Spinal
Dysraphism

Spinal Dysraphism

Spina Bifida Occulta

C. C. Michael James
PhD(Edin), FRCS(Edin)

Orthopaedic Surgeon: W. J. Sanderson Orthopaedic Hospital, Newcastle upon Tyne and Newcastle General Hospital; Clinical Lecturer in the University of Newcastle upon Tyne

L. P. Lassman
MB, BS(Lond), FRCS

Neurological Surgeon: Regional Neurological Centre, Newcastle General Hospital and Royal Victoria Infirmary, Newcastle upon Tyne; Clinical Lecturer in the University of Newcastle upon Tyne

London: Butterworths

ENGLAND: BUTTERWORTH & CO. (PUBLISHERS) LTD.
LONDON: 88 Kingsway, WC2B 6AB

AUSTRALIA: BUTTERWORTH & CO. (AUSTRALIA) LTD.
SYDNEY: 586 Pacific Highway, 2067
MELBOURNE: 343 Little Collins Street, 3000
BRISBANE: 240 Queen Street, 4000

CANADA: BUTTERWORTH & CO. (CANADA) LTD.
TORONTO: 14 Curity Avenue, 374

NEW ZEALAND: BUTTERWORTH & CO. (NEW ZEALAND) LTD.
WELLINGTON: 26–28 Waring Taylor Street, 1

SOUTH AFRICA: BUTTERWORTH & CO.(SOUTH AFRICA)(PTY)LTD.
DURBAN: 152–154 Gale Street

Suggested U.D.C. No. 616·711·7–007·254

ISBN 0 407 39870 8

Printed in Great Britain by
William Clowes & Sons, Limited
London, Beccles and Colchester

Contents

Illustrations

Copyright of all illustrations in this book is held by the University of Newcastle upon Tyne. Permission to reproduce them is gratefully acknowledged.

The colour illustrations have been printed from the plates used in *The Journal of Bone and Joint Surgery* (1962) **44B**, 828.

Some of the monotone illustrations have also previously appeared, as follows:

Archives of Diseases in Childhood (1960) **35**, 315: *Figure 4 (a, b, c)*; (1964) **39**, 125: *Figures 11.5, 11.7, 11.8.*

Journal of Bone and Joint Surgery (1962) **44B**, 828: *Figures 11.4a, 15.12, 19.1.*

Journal of Neurology, Neurosurgery and Psychiatry (1967) **30**, 174: *Figures 15.1, 15.4.*

Paraplegia (1964) **2**, 96: *Figure 15.3.*

Physiotherapy (1962) **48**, 154: *Figures 4.1 (a, b, c), 15.2.*

Psychiatria, Neurologia, Neurochirurgia (1967) **70**, 453: *Figure 11.2.*

Foreword

The problem of spina bifida is one of great topical interest. Controversy continues to rage upon the question as to whether or not all overt cases should be treated by early closure within the first few hours or days of life; despite the conflicts between those who hold different views upon this topic, there can be no doubt that society is likely to be faced with an increasing problem in arranging for the long-term care of those infants saved by operation who would in the past have died within the first year or two of life. While this topic has had considerable publicity of late, relatively little attention has been paid to those forms of malformation of the neuraxis which are less overt and dramatic in their effects but which may be associated with occult spina bifida. Over the last fifteen years, Mr. James and Mr. Lassman have published a series of authoritative papers on spinal dysraphism in all its forms, and in this monograph they now summarize and synthesize their experience. They show very clearly that many spinal dysraphic syndromes have gone unrecognized in the past and that some may be progressively disabling if untreated, while operative treatment carried out sufficiently early may greatly limit or even prevent such disability.

This monograph is logically arranged and succinctly presented. The authors not only review the embryology and anatomy of these malformations, but also report some morbid anatomical studies of their own, as well as discussing radiological and clinical differential diagnosis, treatment and follow-up findings. Dr. Douglas Whitby contributes a useful chapter on anaesthetic techniques used during the myelographic examination of such cases and during operation. The hundred cases which Mr. James and Mr. Lassman have chosen to analyse in detail in this work represent most, if not all, of the dysraphic anomalies which have been previously described. Their clinical analysis is careful, their description of radiological and surgical findings comprehensive and their analysis of the results is completely frank. Clearly operation is only rarely curative, but there is good evidence to indicate that it often prevents increasing disability from developing.

By presenting in this short monograph a summary of their work on spinal dysraphism carried out over the last fifteen years, the authors have done the profession a valuable service. This book will be of interest to all neurologists, neurosurgeons, paediatricians and orthopaedic surgeons, and indeed it deserves to be brought to the attention of all those who are directly or indirectly concerned with the investigation and management of crippling disorders of childhood.

Newcastle upon Tyne   JOHN N. WALTON

PART I

General Considerations

1—Introduction

We started intensive work in this field of spinal dysraphism because spina bifida occulta obtruded as a clinical entity of some importance in the course of a widespread and busy practice in paediatric orthopaedics. It became a subject of urgency because its spinal surgical management had a very bad reputation, and because the patients, being children, were developing more severe disabilities without the apparent possibility of treatment of the primary condition. The time factor, as regards both the children and the other work to be done by the clinicians, precluded extensive preliminary study of the literature, so that it was necessary to proceed in ways which our training and experience suggested to be correct. Many of the children presented in the orthopaedic clinics at a very early stage of the developing disability before a diagnosis could be established so that in due course, when the cause was evident, surgical treatment to prevent further deterioration was still possible. During this period, a clinical syndrome became apparent, and this was described in our publication of 1960 based on work in previous years. This paper was entitled *Spinal Dysraphism* because, although we were principally concerned with the neglected subject of spina bifida occulta, we could not be sure at the time that this was the only type of case which would develop this kind of syndrome. Our caution was justified because it was found that the syndrome is associated with a number of other abnormalities affecting the spinal cord, such as cases which have had a myelomeningocele excised in infancy or early childhood and which have afterwards developed a progressive neurological deficit as a complication, sometimes years later.

Lichtenstein (1940) used the same title to draw attention to cases where the dysraphic state is manifested solely in the spinal cord. He pointed out that the defective fusion of tissues in the dorsal midline of the embryo was 'adequately designated by the term dysraphism or status dysraphicus' (Henneberg, cited by Bremer, 1926).

3

We have continued to work in this field ever since, and have kept detailed records of our cases. Presented here is an account of our experience dealing with the first hundred cases. Our object is to provide a reference book in the hope that, by collecting all this information in one place, help may be given to other workers to make an early diagnosis and to discover better means of investigation and treatment, particularly directed to assessing which cases will benefit by surgery and which will not. The very early case will be seen only in clinics for preventive medicine of children, so it is necessary for clinicians in hospital out-patient departments and polyclinics to recognize the later stages before the spinal cord damage is too severe for surgery to benefit the patient. Urologists and gynaecologists must also be aware of the possibility that a minority of their cases with deficient bladder control will have spina bifida, and that spinal cord surgery is more likely to be beneficial if it is done early and before attempts are made to improve control by urological surgical means.

When the research was started, one of the sources which gave great help was *Spina Bifida and Cranium Bifidum* by Ingraham and his colleagues (1944); a comprehensive survey which included a bibliography covering about 5,000 items published between 1556 and 1943. The amount of literature published since then is considerable, but has been concerned for the most part with small numbers of particular types of abnormality published under a multiplicity of titles. We have undoubtedly been much influenced by what we have read, but are aware that our knowledge of work written in languages other than English is scant; the works and bibliographies of Tridon (1959), of Baruffaldi and Divano (1959) and of Schlegel (1964) have made us very conscious of this. No attempt has been made to annotate all this information; we have noted only those references in each chapter which appear to be relevant to our particular material and which themselves give references to the work of others.

This monograph is arranged in two parts. The first deals with embryology and pathology, clinical aspects, methods of investigation and treatment; the second part is a detailed analysis of all the information we have obtained from our first one hundred cases of spina bifida occulta submitted to laminectomy between April 1957 and June 1965. The majority had clinical abnormalities affecting one or both lower limbs with or without incontinence; some had incontinence alone. There are also some cases with no clinical abnormality but with external cutaneous manifestations on the back. A number of these cases have previously been referred to in separate publications (James and Lassman, 1958, 1960, 1962a, 1962b, 1964; Lassman and James, 1963, 1964, 1967). The forms of clinical abnormalities are described in Chapter 4.

Although this series is consecutive, cases of anterior spina bifida and of spina bifida aperta which proved at operation to have herniation of the meninges and neural tissue outside the vertebral canal, have been excluded. However, one case which had a minute meningocele concealed within a lumbosacral lipoma (Case 15) has been included. For a long time we have believed that minor defects of the spinous process of Sv1 are rarely associated with a surgically remediable abnormality affecting the spinal cord. Therefore 3 further cases of spina bifida occulta which had a minimal laminal defect at Sv1 only have also been excluded; 2 were early cases operated on before the new myelography technique introduced by Gryspeerdt (1963) enabled the conus medullaris to be located; lumbosacral laminectomy in these cases proved negative. One of these 2 patients subsequently developed bilateral foot abnormalities and proved to be a case of Roussy–Levy syndrome while the other remains unilaterally affected and undiagnosed. The third patient was known to have a conus medullaris at the normal level but had continuing sepsis and trophic ulceration in the right foot which was becoming progressively more deformed. Operation was performed because of the progressive nature of the condition and to make sure that we were not incorrect in our opinions about the significance of the position of the conus medullaris and of the minimal laminal defects in relation to surgically treatable abnormalities. In the event, a small brown tumour was found in the right cauda equina which was in continuity with one nerve root, but involved the other roots in adhesions which could not be freed; this tumour was probably an ectopic dorsal root ganglion. The patient's foot has subsequently been operated on, firstly to amputate all the toes and secondly to stabilize it and make it plantigrade.

The majority of the cases were children aged between 8 months and 13½ years; 63 girls and 25 boys. There were 12 adults (including 2 men) aged between 16 and 44 years. The predominance of females is remarkable considering that the distribution between the sexes in spina bifida cystica is about equal.

All these cases have been assessed clinically and have been radiographed to demonstrate laminal defects. They have been investigated further by myelography and submitted to exploration of the spinal cord by laminectomy. Laminectomy is only indicated when the following criteria are present.

(1) Progressive foot deformity with or without neurological deficit; or

(2) incontinence.

(3) The presence of laminal defects of a greater degree than a simple split in the spinous process of Sv1 unless there is associated abnormal widening of the vertebral canal (interpedicular distance).

(4) Myelographic evidence of abnormality or a low situation of the conus medullaris.

Exceptions to the foregoing are a dermal fistula or discharging sinus and a lumbosacral lipoma in either of which exploratory operation is indicated as a preventive measure (Chapter 15).

ACKNOWLEDGEMENTS

We express our gratitude particularly to our collaborators, to Dr. G. L. Gryspeerdt whose skill in radiology produced new diagnostic techniques which have contributed so much to our work, and to Dr. J. D. Whitby who has given the anaesthetics which have made surgery a minimal risk; each of them has made an essential contribution to this monograph.

We also owe much to Sister C. Palfreyman who has nursed the majority of our child patients with such good effect, to Mr. R. W. Ridley and Mrs. P. Bone of the Department of Medical Photography of the University of Newcastle upon Tyne, whose photographs have provided such clear evidence of the spinal anomalies we have found, and to the secretaries who have enabled our records to be kept in order: Miss E. M. Copeland, Miss D. Busby, Miss P. Riddell who managed to cope at the beginning of our research while still doing their own official work, and our two Research Secretaries, Miss S. McVitie and Mrs. A. B. Linkleter, who carried on and finally helped to produce this monograph.

We thank Professor B. E. Tomlinson who has reported on the histological appearances of the tissue obtained at operations and given us much helpful advice; and the many doctors who have sent us the patients.

Mrs. Myra Lassman has given invaluable assistance with proof reading and the preparation of the index, and the late Dr. Muriel M. Johnstone (Mrs. James) designed the summary cards which have been the basis of our documentary system and the means of co-ordinating information.

Our work has been greatly helped by financial support from the Medical Research Council in 1963 and continuously thereafter by the Scientific and Research Committee of the Newcastle Regional Hospital Board.

REFERENCES

Baruffaldi, O. and Divano, N. (1959). *La Spina Bifida*. Padua; Cedam

Bremer, F. W. (1926). 'Klinische Untersuchungen zur Aetiologie der Syringomyelie der Status dysraphicus.' *Dt. Z. NervHeilk*. **95**, 1

Gryspeerdt, G. L. (1963). Myelographic Assessment of Occult Forms of Spinal Dysraphism. *Acta radiol*. **1**, 702

Ingraham, F. D. (1944). *Spina Bifida and Cranium Bifidum. The Children's Hospital, Boston.* Cambridge, Mass; Harvard Univ. Press

James, C. C. M. and Lassman, L. P. (1958). 'Diastematomyelia.' *Archs. Dis. Childh*. **33**, 536

— — (1960). 'Spinal Dysraphism. An Orthopaedic Syndrome in Children Accompanying Occult Forms.' *Archs. Dis. Child*. **35**, 315

— — (1962a). 'Spinal Dysraphism. The Diagnosis and Treatment of Progressive Lesions in Spina Bifida Occulta.' *J. Bone Jt. Surg*. **44B**, 828

— — (1962b). 'Spinal Dysraphism. Spinal Cord Lesions Associated with Spina Bifida Occulta.' *Physiotherapy* **48**, 154

— — (1964). 'Diastematomyelia. A Critical Survey of 24 Cases Submitted to Laminectomy.' *Archs. Dis. Childh*. **39**, 125

Lassman, L. P. and James, C. C. M. (1963). *Lumbosacral Lipomata and Lesions of the Conus Medullaris and Cauda Equina*. Int. Cong. Series, No. 60, pp. 139–141. Amsterdam; Excerpta Medica

— — (1964). 'Spina Bifida Cystica and Occulta; Some Aspects of Spinal Dysraphism.' *Paraplegia* **2**, 96

— — (1967). 'Lumbosacral Lipomas: Critical Survey of 26 Cases Submitted to Laminectomy.' *J. Neurol. Neurosurg. Psychiat*. **30**, 174

Lichtenstein, B. W. (1940). 'Spinal Dysraphism. Spina Bifida and Myelodysplasia.' *Archs. Neurol. Psychiat. Chicago* **44**, 792

Schlegel, K-F. (1964). 'Spina Bifida Occulta und Klauenhohlfuss.' *Ergebn. Chir. Orthop*. **46**, 268

Tridon, P. (1959). *Les Dysraphies de L'Axe Nerveux et de ses Enveloppes Cranio-Rachidiennes. Etude Critique du Status Dysraphicus.* Paris; Doin

2—Embryology and Pathology

Spinal dysraphism is a term revived by Lichtenstein (1940) referring to all forms of developmental abnormality occurring in the midline of the back. There is failure of complete formation of the midline of the future dorsum of the embryo which may affect all or only some of the primary embryonic layers to a greater or lesser degree, varying from case to case, so that there may be abnormalities of the skin, of the muscles, of the blood vessels, of the bones and of the nervous tissues. Spinal dysraphism therefore includes all forms of spina bifida—occulta, aperta, anterior and posterior. Table 2.1 is an adaptation of Lichtenstein's exposition.

TABLE 2.1

SPINA BIFIDA, SPINAL DYSRAPHISM OR THE SPINAL DYSRAPHIC STATE

Adapted from Lichtenstein (1940)

Embryonal origin	Type of dysplasia	Resultant condition
Cutaneous: somatic ectodermal	Cutaneous	Cutaneous defect Hypertrichosis Naevus Dermal sinus
Mesodermal	Vertebral	Split in spinous process Laminal defects Rachischisis
	Dural	Non-fusion of dura mater
Neural: neurectodermal	Neural tube	Myelodysplasia Intramedullary and extra-medullary growths associated with dysraphia
	Neural crest	Ectopia of spinal ganglia and of posterior nerve roots

8

In spina bifida occulta the failure of normal development is not gross, the most severe cases are those which appear to be minor variants of spina bifida aperta where a myelomeningocele or a meningocele has almost formed, the nerve roots or spinal cord are fixed to the dura mater and by a continuous fibrous connection are attached to the skin. The less severe cases are associated with bands running from the spinous processes through the dura mater to the nervous tissue within the theca. These bands are sometimes aberrant posterior nerve roots, sometimes fibrous and sometimes obliterated meningeal extensions. All these anomalies are normally associated with fat deposits, sometimes subcutaneous (as in lumbosacral lipomas), commonly in the defects in the bone of the neural arches and spinous processes and sometimes within the theca. There may also be dermoid tumours as well, sometimes at laminal level and sometimes within the theca either intramedullary or extramedullary.

The basic clinical differences between spina bifida aperta and spina bifida occulta result from the nature of their origin. Spina bifida aperta is essentially a developmental failure of the tissues of the spinal cord itself, complicated by the destructive process *in utero* described by Warkany, Wilson and Geiger (1958), who observed degenerative changes, abnormal vascularization, haemorrhages and round-cell infiltration in the neural plate of rat embryos in increasing amounts with advancing gestational age. Also, there is the cellular hyperplasia described by Patten (1953) and the factors affecting the brain with probable secondary effects on the spinal cord.

In spina bifida occulta, in contrast, there may be dysplasia of the spinal cord, but of small degree, which is not accompanied by similar destructive action, nor by brain anomalies, as far as is known at present.

For our clinical purposes to differentiate between the occult and overt forms of spina bifida we have had to rely on the macroscopic evidence yielded by surgical exploration. Where there has been herniation of the meninges outside the vertebral canal, with or without neural content, the case has been classified as 'aperta'; where there is no such herniation the case has been classed as one of 'occulta'. This differentiation is that of Koch. Our own cases illustrate the gradation from spina bifida aperta to spina bifida occulta very well (Lassman and James, 1964).

The clinical importance of spina bifida occulta lies in the extrinsic anomalies which bind down the spinal cord or its nerve roots and prevent them from changing their position within the vertebral canal as they normally should to accommodate to the growth of the vertebral column and of the spinal cord. If the spinal cord is tethered

9

it will suffer a traction force during vertebral growth which it can accommodate to some degree in some cases by increasing its own rate of growth, but when this compensatory reaction can do no more, the traction force will cause failure of neuronal conduction and ischaemia owing to failure of blood supply or to venous congestion with possible thrombosis. The fat and fibrous tissue, which so commonly occur in association with frustration of development of embryonic tissues, further complicates matters by increasing in bulk and thus causing pressure. It is all these factors which produce the changes in the lower limbs, bladder and bowel. Consequently it is essential to recognize the early clinical evidence so that the extrinsic structures can be removed before they can produce irreversible damage to the nervous tissue.

EMBRYOLOGY

In its very early stages the embryonic disc is two layers thick; the ectoderm on the future dorsal aspect has the amniotic cavity on one side and endoderm ventrally, forming the roof of the yolk sac (day 12). At the cranial end of the disc, these two layers form the prochordal plate and caudally the ectoderm forms the primitive streak. At the cranial end of the latter, adjacent to the embryonic disc, the cells thicken to form the primitive knot (Hensen's node) in the centre of which an inward movement of cells results in the formation of a pit, the primitive pit, which is equivalent to the blastopore. From this pit, cells migrate cranially in the midline between ectoderm and endoderm to form the notochordal process which grows to meet the prochordal plate. Following this, cells migrate from the sides of the primitive streak forwards on each side of the notochord to separate ectoderm and endoderm except at the prochordal plate around which they pass; these cells constitute the third embryonic layer, the mesoderm (day 18).

The pit in the blastopore deepens within the notochordal process which becomes tubular and fuses with the endoderm in the roof of the yolk sac. Openings appear in the floor of the process which is now the notochordal or neurenteric (amnioenteric) canal whose other extremity already opens into the amniotic cavity so that there is now a direct communication between the latter and the yolk sac. The openings in the floor of the notochordal canal join together so that the notochordal process becomes a groove in the roof of the yolk sac, but gradually the endoderm on each side grows together in the midline to reform the yolk sac roof; the notochordal process by the folding together of its lateral margins forms a tube, the *definitive*

10

notochord, to lie once more between endoderm and ectoderm (completed by the end of 4 weeks, 4 mm, about 25 somite stage). The *neural plate*, ultimately to become the brain and spinal cord, is formed by the ectoderm, cranial to the primitive knot, and to begin with, on each side of the notochord. The neural plate sinks inwards in the midline, becoming grooved and its lateral margins curl over to join in the dorsal midline to form the neural tube (starts with somites 4–6 at 7 somite stage, 21 days). The tube grows cranially to form the brain and caudally to form the spinal cord; the tube openings, the anterior and posterior neuropores, close at the 20 somite and 25 somite stages respectively. The *neural crest* cells develop at the margins of the neural plate and separate from it before the tube is completed and also separate from the cutaneous ectoderm which was previously the sheet of ectoderm continuous laterally with the neural plate. The two lateral sheets of cutaneous ectoderm come together in the midline separating from and lying superficial to the neural tube as it is completed. Ultimately the human embyro develops 42–44 somites.

The foregoing is based on the account given by Hamilton, Boyd and Mossman (1962) and it is difficult to discover from books on descriptive embryology how the caudal part of the spinal cord is formed. Holmdahl (1933) divided spinal cord development into two parts; the cranial end as described above and the caudal part, in the embryonic tail, from the pluripotential cells of the primitive streak. Unfortunately, he does not detail the nature of the junction between the two, nor the site in relation to the vertebral bodies except that he suggests that it occurs in the middle of the rump but states that the lumbar and sacral spine together with the axial organs at and below this level are all formed from primitive streak material.

According to Hamilton, Boyd and Mossman, at somite 1 stage the neural plate tapers away caudally on each side of the primitive streak and as the embryonic disc lengthens the neural plate extends caudally so that the primitive pit (blastopore) comes to lie within it. The existence of the neurenteric canal is short and the time at which it ceases to open into the amniotic sac is not stated. From the work of Kunitomo (1918) one concludes that the primitive pit associated with the formation of the notochord no longer exists at the 4 mm stage (25–28 somites) since the notochord and the neural tube in his specimens both end in the tail by merging with the mesodermic cell-mass associated with the remains of the primitive streak material.

Writers dealing with developmental anomalies vary in their descriptions of the development of the spinal cord in the tail. Some

11

state that it develops as a rod which canalizes secondarily, others suggest that it continues to be produced from each side of the primitive knot (Hensen's node) which is the thickened area at the cranial margin of the primitive streak, thus developing two parallel neural plates, which unite as a tube in a manner which seems to resemble the tail development of the tadpole (Jenkinson, 1925). None of these writers names any authority for his statement so that the true situation is obscure. Gruenwald (1941) states firmly that caudal levels of the spinal cord differentiate as a primarily solid cord from the trunk-tail node and continues that there is 'ignorance of the processes of distribution and determination of material going on in the trunk-tail node before visible differentiation'. Holmdahl (1933) suggests similarly that the neural tube is secondarily canalized and stresses that the relation of the cutaneous ectoderm to the neural tube in the caudal area is quite different from the developmental relationship cranially. He points out that cranially, the cutaneous ectoderm is continuous with the lateral margins of the neural plate and that as the latter folds to form a tube the ectoderm is drawn into the midline to unite there and relinquish its contact with neural tissue; in the tail region, however, the cutaneous ectoderm is formed quite separately and grows medially over the neural tissue without having any direct contact. The second form of development is unlike the first which in its earliest stages has three embryonic layers, because it emerges from the pluripotential cells of the primitive streak where the embryonic layers do not exist. Hamilton, Boyd and Mossman, however, state that the primitive streak cannot be regarded as a special centre of proliferation but it is possible that this statement refers only to the earliest stages of embryonic layer formation. According to Orts Llorca (1934), quoted by Gruenwald (1941), the neural crests develop by outgrowth from the dorsal portion of the neural tube caudal to somite 24 and further caudally (somites 31–35), arise partly or entirely from the ventral part of the neural tube. The neural crest cells provide material for many structures throughout the body but they also develop into the posterior root ganglia from which nerve fibres grow into the spinal cord from out-side it to connect with the cells of the posterior horns.

Kunitomo's longest specimen in terms of somite formation was 11 mm with 38 primitive vertebrae (about day 37), the last being larger than the thirty-seventh and thirty-sixth by inclusion of material from the mesodermic remnant (of the primitive streak material) which had been converted into a non-vertebrated tail. His diagram shows that the neural tube and notochord reach to the end of this tail. At this stage both he and Streeter (1919) detect the beginning of formation of the filum terminale by dedifferentiation of the neural tube which shows a change at 32 vertebral level at which point the wide canal cranially, with thick walls and mantle and marginal zones, narrows caudally to a more slender part with a narrow canal and walls of ependymal zone only. The formation of the neural tube is completed at this stage and developing into the finite spinal cord and filum terminale.

During the process of dedifferentiation of the neural tube to form the filum terminale the canal narrows and becomes divided into several parts, each containing a cavity; these gradually disappear and at the 67 mm stage the filum terminale completely disappears caudal to the thirty-second vertebra. At the upper border of the twenty-seventh vertebra the dura mater leaves the wall of the vertebral canal, forming a sheath reaching the filum terminale between the twenty-eighth and twenty-ninth vertebrae. The caudal end of the dural sac recedes cranial-ward with growth. The filum terminale increases in length during development, partly by actual growth and partly by addition from the receding conus medullaris; its original most caudal part (the coccygeal medullary vestige) merges into the caudal ligament which is formed from distal atrophic scleromeres. The second coccygeal vertebra and those caudal to it in the adult represent the remains of a true tail.

The conus medullaris can be detected (Kunitomo) at the 39 mm stage below 34 vertebra and at the 50 mm stage it is at about 30/31 vertebra level. From this point it ascends within the vertebral canal as a result of differential growth rates of vertebral column and spinal cord so that at 25 weeks (Streeter) it is at Sv1 level, at birth at Lv3 and at completion of growth it is in the region of the disc between Lv1 and Lv2.

The dura mater is formed and separates from the vertebral rudiments between days 30 and 42; at about day 47 (27–31 mm) it can be traced all around the inner wall of the vertebral canal particularly in the thoracic region (Sensenig, 1951). Pia mater is differentiated from spinal cord at about the same time but arachnoid mater which is delaminated from dura mater late in foetal life is not evident before the 80 mm stage and is insufficiently separated until after birth to form the subdural space although Kunitomo states that all three meningeal tissues are evident at 67 mm.

DISCUSSION

The lack of information about the normal embryology of the tail-bud prevents our drawing any conclusions about the developmental

13

nature of the abnormalities which we have found at operation (Chapter 11 *et seq.*), we can only draw attention to the theories put forward by others. If Holmdahl's (1933) description of spinal cord development is correct as occurring in two forms, the method of union between them is important as also is its site in terms of vertebral level. Spina bifida aperta which so commonly occurs in the lumbar and sacral regions could well be associated with defective union of the two forms. Defects occurring at points of union of developing tissues are well known in other parts of the body. Von Recklinghausen (1886) gave his opinion that spina bifida aperta resulted from a primary defect of development of the blastoderm and was not caused secondarily and, apart from Gardner (1968) and Barry, Patten and Stewart (1957), other theorists seem to agree with von Recklinghausen. Lemire, Shephard and Alvord (1965) have an interesting discussion on the pathogenesis of myelomeningoceles particularly relating to the theories of Gardner and of Barry and his colleagues and put forward a theory of defect in the development of the limiting membrane as being part of the pathology; Gardner's later work (1968) answers these criticisms. A most comprehensive survey is provided by Källén (1968) and readers are referred to the original article. Källén discusses experimental work including inductive mechanisms and the theories mentioned above.

Gardner's theory (1968) is based on the existence of hydrocephalus and hydromyelia as a normal condition in early embryonic life as a result of fluid secreted by the neuroepithelium in the first place and later by the choroid plexus. He postulates that by preventing the normal circulation of cerebrospinal fluid, delay or failure of permeation of the roof of the fourth ventricle will produce all grades of the abnormalities encountered in dysraphic states from syringomyelia, Chiari malformations and diastematomyelia to myelocele. With the development of normal permeation of the rhombic roof the subarachnoid spaces are dissected open but if there is delay in this process, the force of the pulsation of the choroid plexuses causes hydrodynamic effects and progressive hydromyelia. Williams (1969) suggests that venous pressure changes also contribute. Since the shape and closure of the vertebral canal are secondary to neural tube and spinal cord development, laminal defects and increased size of the vertebral canal are accounted for, as well as elements of vertebral body abnormality. Gardner describes four stages of hydromyelia, the first is associated with a transient degree of over-distension leading to a normal central canal of the spinal cord and enlargement of the vertebral canal. There may be failure of fusion of the vertebral arches. Syringomyelia may appear in adult life. The second stage is likely to produce diastematomyelia but Gardner here states that the two hemicords are likely to have mesodermal tissue intervening which in its least degree will form a septum of arachnoid. We have never seen a septum which did not include dura mater, although we have found what we have described as veils of arachnoid within a single dural tube associated with diastematomyelia but these did not constitute a septum dividing the compartments: this is a minor point of semantics. Stage three produces a meningocele because the internal hydromyelia becomes external and the expanding subarachnoid space bulges beneath cutaneous ectoderm. This theory of dissection of the subarachnoid space is not entirely compatible with the findings of Sensenig and Kunitomo noted on p. 13. Stage four produces a myelocele by forcible rupture of the roof plate and cutaneous ectoderm; Gardner here refutes von Recklinghausen (1886) who considered that myelocele was primary and not secondary. The theory also logically accounts for all three types of the malformation of the brain described by Chiari and the reader is referred to the original article which while considering the theories of other workers, gives a detailed, clear and reasonable exposition of the whole subject of the developmental aspects of spina bifida and cranium bifidum.

Barry, Patten and Stewart (1957) developing the theme of over-growth (in a morphological sense) of neural plate tissue described by Patten (1953) ascribe myelocele formation to prevention of closure of the neural tube by this tissue overgrowth which is also found to a lesser degree in the normally formed spinal cord cephalad to the myelocele as determined by external measurement. Overgrowth of tissue in the brain, as similarly determined by external comparison of brain size in embryos, is given as the cause of the Arnold–Chiari malformation which results in blockage of the subarachnoid space at the level of the foramen magnum and the production of secondary hydrocephalus. Barry and colleagues refute the suggestion that the overgrowth of neural plate tissue in a myelocele is occurring second-arily at a point where the neural tube has failed to close because, they say, the overgrowth is not limited to the area of the myelocele, it also occurs in the developed spinal cord cephalad to the myelocele as inferred from the increase in volume of these segments and again in the brain as mentioned above. They do not produce direct evidence of actual cellular overgrowth in these other areas nor does Patten (1953) in this original description of overgrowth. Emery and Naik (1968) have not been able to demonstrate tissue overgrowth in human morbid anatomy studies.

Barry, Patten and Stewart (1957) also cite a case where there was diastematomyelia but only a single notochord. They suggest that this is due to a degree of overgrowth of the neural folds sufficient to distort but not to prevent their fusion. Our P.M. Case 137 also had a single notochord (p. 23).

The final theory to be considered here is that of Bentley and Smith (1960) who in describing and naming the split-notochord syndrome have drawn together information from separate previous authors, principally Saunders (1943), McLetchie, Purves and Saunders (1954) and Bremer (1952) and correlated these with their own observations. In essence they postulate that, for reasons unknown, the notochord develops in duplicate in part of its extent leaving temporarily or permanently a persistent neurenteric canal connecting the embryonic gut with the dorsal surface of the embryo. The canal may become sealed off in embryonic life leaving endodermal, mesodermal and ectodermal rests within the tissues surrounding them. Since these rests are isolated early in embryonic life their final situation at the end of foetal growth will be distant from their earlier relationships. The theory accounts for a variety of vertebral and cranial anomalies: prevertebral cysts, intestinal duplications and fissures: and post-vertebral cysts, epidermoids, teratomas and sinuses. It will also account for diastematomyelia and both anterior and posterior meningoceles. If the whole canal remains patent the abnormalities are usually incompatible with life but occasionally infants are born with enteric fistulae presenting on the back.

If more were known about the embryology of the tail-bud, it might be possible to explain the formation of the frustrated meningo-celes which we have termed meningocele manqué (Chapter 14) and which are so commonly found on surgical exploration in the lumbo-sacral region. Gardner's is the best theory to account for this condition as being the result of a combination of internal and external hydromyelia which has become compensated early on.

REFERENCES

Barry, A., Patten, B. M. and Stewart, B. H. (1957). 'Possible Factors in the Development of the Arnold–Chiari Malformation.' *J. Neurosurg.* **14**, 285

Bentley, J. F. R. and Smith, J. R. (1960). 'Developmental Posterior Enteric Remnants and Spinal Malformations.' *Archs. Dis. Childh.* **35**, 76

Bremer, J. L. (1952). 'Dorsal Intestinal Fistula; Accessory Neurenteric Canal; Diastematomyelia.' *Archs. Path.* **54**, 132

Emery, J. L. and Naik, D. R. (1968). 'Spinal Cord Segment Lengths in Children with Meningomyelocele and the "Cleland–Arnold–Chiari" Malformation.' *Br. J. Radiol.* **41**, 287

Gardner, W. J. (1968). 'Myelocele: Rupture of the Neural Tube?' In *Clinical Neurology*, pp. 57–59. Proceedings of the Congress of Neurological Surgeons, San Francisco, 1967. Baltimore; Williams and Wilkins

Gruenwald, P. (1941). 'Tissue Anomalies of Probable Neural Crest Origin in a 20 mm Human Embryo with Myeloschisis.' *Archs. Path.* **31**, 489

Hamilton, W. J., Boyd, J. D. and Mossman, H. W. (1962). *Human Embryology*. 3rd Edition. Cambridge; Heffer

Holmdahl, D. E. (1933). 'Die Zweifache Bildungsweise des Zentralen Nerven Systems bei den Wirbeltieren.' *Arch. EntwMech. Org.* **129**, 206

Jenkinson, J. W. (1925). *Vertebrate Embryology*, p. 155. London; Oxford University Press

Källén, B. (1968). 'Early Embryogenesis of the Central Nervous System with Special Reference to Closure Defects.' *Devl. Med. Child Neurol.* Suppl. **16**, 44

Kunitomo, K. (1918). 'The Development and Reduction of the Tail and of the Caudal End of the Spinal Cord.' *Contr. Embryol.* **8**, 161

Lassman, L. P. and James, C. C. M. (1964). 'Spina Bifida Cystica and Occulta; Some Aspects of Spinal Dysraphism.' *Paraplegia* **2**, 96

Lemire, R. J., Shephard, T. H. and Alvord, E. C. Jr. (1965). 'Caudal Myeloschisis (Lumbosacral) Spina Bifida Cystica in a five millimeter (Horizon XIV) Human Embryo.' *Anat. Rec.* **152**, 9

Lichtenstein, B. W. (1940). 'Spinal Dysraphism. Spina Bifida and Myelodysplasia.' *Archs. Neurol. Psychiat.* **44**, 792

McLetchie, N. G. B., Purves, J. K. and Saunders, R. L. de C. H. (1954). 'The Genesis of Gastric and Certain Intestinal Diverticula and Enterogenous Cysts.' *Surgery Gynec. Obstet.* **99**, 135

Orts Llorca, F. (1934). *Z. Anat. EntwGesch.* **102**, 462

Patten, Bradley, M. (1953). 'Embryological Stages in the Establishing of Myeloschisis with Spina Bifida.' *Am. J. Anat.* **93**, 365

Recklinghausen, F. von (1886). 'Untersuchungen uber die Spina bifida.' *Virchows Arch. path. Anat. Physiol.* **105**, 243 and 373

Saunders, R. L. de C. H. (1943). 'Combined Anterior and Posterior Spina Bifida in a Living Neonatal Human Female.' *Anat. Rec.* **87**, 255

Sensenig, E. C. (1951). 'The Early Development of the Meninges of the Spinal Cord in Human Embryos.' *Contr. Embryol.* **34**, 147

Streeter, G. L. (1919). 'Factors Involved in the Formation of the Filum Terminale.' *Am. J. Anat.* **25**, 1

Warkany, J., Wilson, J. G. and Geiger, J. F. (1958). 'Myeloschisis and Myelomeningocele Produced Experimentally in the Rat.' *J. comp. Neurol.* **109**, 35

Williams, B. (1969). 'The Distending Force in the Production of Communicating Syringomyelia.' *Lancet* **2**, 189

3—Morbid Anatomy Research

After clinical work was started on children with spina bifida occulta, it was found that the conus medullaris was usually situated very low in the vertebral canal and that there was no published information about its change in position between birth and full growth so that it was not known if these levels were abnormal. Streeter (1919) had shown that on average the conus medullaris lies at the level of Lv3 body at birth and is at about the level of the intervertebral disc between Lv1 and Lv2 in adult life. Furthermore we were unaware whether the extrinsic abnormalities of the spinal cord, found at operation, were always associated with laminal defects or not, nor was it known with what degree of laminal defect they usually occurred. One of us therefore started an elaborate investigation in the postmortem room of the Newcastle General Hospital. The intention was to radiograph every adult body passing through the mortuary to determine the incidence of laminal defects, and to perform autopsies to discover the state of the spinal cord and the level of the conus medullaris whether there were laminal defects or not. It was further intended to perform autopsies on all children passing through the department for the same purposes. Since the laminae are not well ossified before the age of 5 years, radiographic examination of these children was not done. In the event, in spite of the encouragement and assistance of the Scientific and Research Committee of the Newcastle Regional Hospital Board which we acknowledge with gratitude, there were considerable handicaps, amongst them absence of consent for autopsy, which prevented the investigation of a large enough sample to produce definitive results within the time available. Nevertheless the information obtained has been a very useful guide in the clinical sphere.

Level of the conus medullaris—Adults
Streeter's findings (1919) about the level of the conus medullaris

were confirmed. Autopsies were performed on 45 adults, 13 of whom had been shown to have laminal defects by radiography, and with the exception of one case (P.M. 137) the spinal cord, cauda equina and filum terminale appeared normal. The levels of the conus medullaris in these 44 normal cases were as follows:

Tv12	*Tv12/Lv1 disc*	*Lv1*	*Lv1/2 disc*	*Lv2*
4	2	20	14	4

Reimann and Anson (1944) reported on their own series of 129 adult specimens and collected from the records of 3 other authors a further 672 cases. In these 801 cases the upper limit of spinal cord termination was Tv12, the lowest limit Lv3; 97·8 per cent terminated at or above the intervertebral disc Lv2/3, and 1·8 per cent over Lv3 so that this level must be regarded as the lowest limit of normality. They comment that Thompson's series of 115 male and 83 female subjects indicate that there was a significant sex difference wherein the mean level for the female group was a vertebral third lower than for male subjects but the range was shorter, the male termination being more variable. Jit and Charnalia (1959) found the same sex variation in their 80 cases (50 male and 30 female): in 20 per cent of female and 10 per cent of male subjects the spinal cord terminated below the upper third of Lv2 but the range of termination was the same for male and female subjects. Our own series, 31 males and 13 females, was too small to allow any conclusions to be drawn.

As regards racial characteristics, Reimann and Anson mention that there was no difference in adult spinal cord termination between whites and Negroes, but in relation to the age of attaining the adult level of termination, Jit and Charnalia quote Rao (1949) as showing a racial difference in that in 15 foetuses Rao found that the adult level was attained at the 214 mm stage. This is an exceptional finding as other authors have agreed with Streeter (1919). Jit and Charnalia comment that there may be racial differences in this respect; they were examining North Indians and Rao was examining South Indians.

Reimann and Anson (1944) excluded from their series a single case of sacral termination of the spinal cord, the only one found in 650 laminectomies. They comment on the effects of low sacral fixation on the lengthening and dislocation of the thoracic and lumbar cord segments. Segments of the spinal medulla measured from 2·4 cm at Tv10 level to 5·4 cm at Lv4. They state that normally no segment of cord below Tv10 is over 2·0 cm long, the segments together from that to the fifth lumbar level being 12·8 cm long. In their specimen the same linear group (Tv10–Lv5) measured 27·0 cm in length. In mentioning 'levels' in this context, we assume they mean segments to be between nerve root origins Tv10–Lv5. This increase in segmental length near the point of fixation agrees with the findings of Barry, Patten and Stewart (1957) and of Emery and Naik (1968) that the tension is dissipated within 4 segments from that point.

Level of the conus medullaris—Children

Autopsies on 25 children without neurological abnormalities and aged between less than one hour and 8 years suggest that the conus medullaris has attained the level of the body of Lv2 by the age of 5 months at the latest (20 cases). At this age the vertebral body is still very small relative to the conus medullaris and it was difficult to be sure whether the conus situation was over the middle of the vertebral body, its upper or its lower border. In 5 more cases, aged 7 and 10 months, 3, 6 and 8 years, the youngest and the 3 oldest children had a conus level of Lv1 lower border but in the child aged 10 months the conus was still at Lv2 level (Table 3.1).

There were similarly mixed findings in 3 further cases of hydrocephalus without spina bifida. In these three children the conus

TABLE 3.1

LEVEL OF THE CONUS MEDULLARIS IN 25 CHILDREN

Birth weight	Age at death	Conus level
9 lb	less than 1 hour	Lv3
7 lb 4 oz	less than 1 hour	Lv1
4 lb 14 oz	3 hours	Lv2
—	4 hours	Lv2/3
3 lb 5 oz	9 hours	Lv3
6 lb 15 oz	20 hours	Lv3
8 lb 0 oz	2 days	Lv3
6 lb 0 oz	2 days	Lv2
5 lb 1 oz	3 days	Lv3
6 lb 3 oz	3 days	Lv2
6 lb 4 oz	4 days	Lv2
—	14 days	Lv1
—	3 weeks	Lv2
—	3 weeks	Lv2
—	5 weeks	Lv2
—	8 weeks	Lv2/3
—	2 months	Lv2
—	2 months	Lv3
—	4 months	Lv2
—	5 months	Lv2
—	7 months	Lv1/2
—	10 months	Lv2
—	3 years	Lv1/2
—	6 years	Lv1/2
—	8 years	Tv12/Lv1

level was Lv2 although they were aged 6 weeks, 6 months and 14 months. The whole series is too small to produce definitive information but we regard a conus level at Lv3 or lower as abnormal over the age of 6 months since we are dealing with clinical cases with abnormal physical signs although Reimann and Anson (1944) have shown that the lowest level of normality in 1·8 per cent is at Lv3.

The conus level was also seen to be unrelated to birth weight in these few cases. A further case, birth weight 2 lb 10 oz, lived only 10 minutes: the conus level was Sv1 but the infant had multiple non-spinal congenital defects: double harelip, cleft palate, horse-shoe kidney with double ureters and heart abnormalities.

Burrows (1968) reports a personal communication from Barson (1967) who examined the normal spinal cords of foetuses and children aged between 13 weeks of gestation and puberty. Barson concluded that the differential in the rates of growth between spinal cord and vertebral column begins at the twelfth week of gestation and that the rate of ascent of the conus medullaris is most rapid from then until the twentieth week, continuing at a slow but steady rate until the adult level of Lv1–2 is attained. The normal spinal cord, *on average*, ends opposite Lv3 at 30 weeks and at Lv2 at 40 weeks, reaching Lv1–2 at about 9 weeks after a full-term gestation. Barson has confirmed with us that this statement is essentially correct and adds that the majority of his 252 normal cases were in the latter half of gestation. His detailed account of this work and the conclusions to be drawn have been published recently (1970).

Incidence of spina bifida

In this research project, an attempt was made to radiograph every body passing through the mortuary to determine the incidence of laminal defects. Out of 1,172 individuals radiographed, such defects were found in 58, an incidence of 5 per cent. There were 10 children aged 6 years to 15 years and 1,162 adults aged 17 to 95 years. Although the series was theoretically unselected, the cases were not representative of the population as a whole as evidenced by the age distribution: 86 per cent male subjects and 88 per cent female subjects were aged between 50 and 95 years. The remaining 14 per cent male and 12 per cent female subjects were aged between 17 and 49 years. Of the total adults of known age and sex in this series 633 were male and 512 female.

There have been several published estimates of the incidence of spina bifida occulta in the population varying between 10 per cent

(Kohler, 1928) and 33 per cent (Roederer and Lagrot, 1926) but our finding is very low indeed and probably relates to the selection of cases for examination.

The area radiographed was the whole lumbar spine and sacrum; laminal defects at Sv3, 4 and 5 have been ignored. Since the majority of laminal defects are known to occur in this area of the vertebral column it is doubtful if the 5 per cent incidence in this series would have been changed very much if the whole spine had been examined. In some cases it was difficult to decide whether there was a defect or not; these have been classed as normal. The distribution of laminal defects amongst the 58 positive findings are shown in Table 3.2.

TABLE 3.2

LOCALIZATION OF LAMINAL DEFECTS FOUND ON RADIOGRAPHY
AND NUMBERS CONFIRMED BY AUTOPSY

Affected laminae	No. of cases	Proved by autopsy
Lv4, 5 and Sv1	1	1 (P.M. Case 137)
Lv5 and Sv1	12	4
Lv5 minimal	1	0
Sv1 major	14	3
Sv1 minimal	25	2
Sv1 and 2	3	1
Sv2	2	2
	58	13

The numbers of cases of each defect examined by autopsy is noted alongside each group; apart from P.M. Case 137, no spinal cord abnormality was found. There were 6 cases of the anomaly described by de Anquin (1959) in which the laminae of Sv1 are absent and its spinous process is a continuation of Lv5.

From the evidence of the adult autopsies, we deduced that surgically treatable congenital abnormalities of the spinal cord, cauda equina or filum terminale were not likely to be found unless the laminal defects were more extensive than those at Sv1 alone and this surmise is supported by 3 cases in life which were submitted to laminectomy (p. 5). These 3 cases were operated on because their clinical state suggested that the spinal cord was abnormal.

Our exceptional case (P.M. 137) mentioned above showed laminal defects at Lv 4/5 and Sv1 and the disc between Lv 3/4 was congenitally narrow. At autopsy, a bone septum was found passing from the mid-line of the laminae of Lv3/4 into a very small hiatus in the meninges; its attenuated deep attachment was to the upper margin of the body of Lv4. There were two dural tubes at the site of the hiatus which completely occupied the gap between the two spinal cords of diastematomyelia. The conus medullaris was immediately caudal to this septum and was situated over Lv4 vertebral body; the dural sac ended at Sv3. The intervertebral discs Lv3/4 and Lv4/5 showed no evidence of abnormality of the nucleus pulposus which might suggest splitting of the notochord. The subject was a woman aged 64 years who had died following a myocardial infarction. On admission to hospital 14 days previously she had had no neurological abnormal-ity; her feet and lower limbs were of equal length and there was no external cutaneous manifestation on the back. There had been no history of urinary infection or frequency. She had had 6 pregnancies with no miscarriages but one child had died of nephrosis. An operation for procidentia had been performed 2 years previously. This case indicates that a septum associated with diastematomyelia will not necessarily cause injury, that the spinal cord has a definite capacity by growth to accommodate itself to fixation and that the theories that neurological damage can result from traction on the spinal cord are not entirely sound. Nevertheless our clinical cases of diastematomyelia indicate that prevention of spinal cord ascent by pressure of a septum can cause local reaction during growth (Cases 14, 52 and 57, p. 65), but only one improved following removal of the offending septum. It is possible that the outcome may be in-fluenced by the site of the septum within the vertebral canal, by its distance from the conus medullaris or by the amount of space in the hiatus of the diastematomyelia for movement during growth; this subject is discusssed further on p. 65 (diastematomyelia) and p. 87 (tight filum terminale) (James and Lassman, 1970).

During the course of this work, an attempt was made to discover how much movement occurred in the spinal cord at the conus medullaris during flexion and extension of the vertebral column. The range was very small at any age, being slightly greater in small children. Barson (1970) working with embryos and neonates states 'the level of the conus medullaris is altered a little by the degree of flexion of the spine'. Reid (1960) examined post-mortem a number of cases aged between 15 and 75 years and was mainly concerned with the effects of cervical spondylosis. He found that between full flexion and full extension the greatest range of movement amounting to a maximum of 1·8 cm was at the levels of the roots of Cv8–Tv5; at Tv10 the full range in 3 subjects was between 2 and 3 mm. With flexion only, in 6 cases the movement at Tv10 varied between 3 mm upward and 1 mm downward and at Tv12 it was between 2 mm upward and 5 mm downward. He also examined segmental stretching in full flexion: this was maximal at Cv3–Cv6 (average 11·3 per cent), at Tv7–Tv11 it averaged 3·2 per cent and at Tv11–Lv1 it was 3·4 per cent; this examination was on 4 subjects aged 15–40 years, 2 male and 2 female.

REFERENCES

De Anquin, C. E. (1959). 'Spina Bifida Occulta with Engagement of the Fifth Lumbar Spinous Process.' *J. Bone Jt. Surg.* **41B**, 486

Barry, A., Patten, B. M. and Stewart, D. H. (1957). 'Possible Factors in the Development of the Arnold–Chiari Malformation.' *J. Neurosurg.* **14**, 285

Barson, A. J. (1970). 'The Vertebral Level of Termination of the Spinal Cord during Normal and Abnormal Development.' *J. Anat.* **106**, 489

Burrows, F. G. O. (1968). 'Some Aspects of Occult Spinal Dysraphism; A Study of 90 Cases.' *Br. J. Radiol.* **41**, 496

Emery, J. L. and Naik, D. (1968). 'Spinal Cord Segment Lengths in Children with Meningomyelocoele and the "Cleland–Arnold–Chiari" Deformity.' *Br. J. Radiol.* **41**, 287

James, C. C. M. and Lassman, L. P. (1970). 'Diastematomyelia and the Tight Filum Terminale.' *J. neurol. Sci.* **10**, 193

Jit, I. and Charnalia, V. M. (1959). 'The Vertebral Level of the Termination of the Spinal Cord.' *J. anat. Soc. India* **8**, 93

Kohler, A. (1928). *Rontgenology. The Borderlands of the Normal and Early Pathological in the Skiagram.* 1st Edition, p. 242. London; Bailliere, Tindall and Cox

Rao, V. S. (1949). 'The Lower Limit of the Spinal Cord in South Indian Foetuses.' *J. Anat.* **83**, 175

Reid, J. D. (1960). 'Effects of Flexion-extension Movements of the Head and Spine upon Spinal Cord and Nerve Roots.' *J. Neurol. Neurosurg. Psychiat.* **23**, 214

Reimann, A. F. and Anson, B. J. (1944). 'Vertebral Level of Termination of the Spinal Cord, with Report of a Case of Sacral Cord.' *Anat. Rec.* **88**, 127

Roederer, C. and Lagrot, F. (1926). 'Le diagnostic radiologique du spina bifida occulta lombosacré.' *J. Radiol. Électrol.* **10**, 255

Streeter, G. L. (1919). 'Factors Involved in the Formation of the Filum Terminale.' *Am. J. Anat.* **25**, 1

4—Syndromes and Clinical Presentation

Occult forms of spinal dysraphism are not commonly evident at birth. At that time, the function of the spinal cord may not be impaired but as the child grows a dysraphic lesion will begin to have an effect by preventing the spinal cord from 'ascending' within the vertebral canal, by pressure from the increasing size of some abnormal tissue such as a lipoma or dermoid or by pressure from normal growth of the spinal cord within a vertebral canal which is abnormally narrowed, for instance, by inversion of laminae. The effect then is a gradual interference with neuronal conduction or local blood supply leading to diminution of sensation and muscle imbalance.

In some cases, the spinal cord is affected *in utero* in which case the infant may be incontinent or have a foot deformity at birth. More commonly the foot deformity is a severe calcaneovalgus but forms of talipes equinovarus also occur; these may be unilateral or bilateral and the two feet may have opposite deformities, that is, one is calcaneovalgus, the other equinovarus. These are, of course, the foot deformities so commonly seen in cases of spina bifida aperta and while not always present at birth in spina bifida occulta they may develop during the course of growth so that the pattern of neurological deficit in the growing child is that of spina bifida aperta but over an extended time-scale. Sixteen children in this series had a history of a foot deformity at birth but it is not possible to identify the types with any accuracy (Chapter 17).

At birth, the back may appear to be normal but 73 of our cases had the external cutaneous manifestations which are associated with spina bifida. Fifty-seven presented with the more easily identifiable hypertrichosis or lipoma and 16 with the less easily recognizable stigmata of naevus, dimple, sinus or a slightly pigmented scarred patch of skin (Chapter 15).

Symptoms

The commonest symptom of late development of neurological deficit is a peculiarity of gait which may occur at any age from 1 to 16 years. The complaint may be of distortion of one shoe, or of poor posture associated with a short leg and sometimes because one foot is found to be shorter than the other. The shoe distortion may result from foot deformity or from the peculiar foot action which occurs in the very earliest stage of neurological deficit.

Pain is not a feature but there is occasionally complaint of metatarsalgia probably resulting from a protective gait. Backache as an initiating symptom has been mentioned by some other authors but has been present in our series in 1 child only and 1 adult, although another adult complained of considerable tenderness in a large naevoid area of the back which gave her a sickening feeling if she were knocked or bumped in that area (Case 74).

One boy aged $2\frac{1}{2}$ years (82) presented with hot-water bottle burns on the toes of one hitherto unsuspected insensitive foot.

Gait

The abnormality of gait, almost imperceptible early on, consists of an elevation of the first metatarsal head as though something like a verruca were underneath it, the great toe usually remaining flexed. Occasionally this is accompanied by adduction movement of the forefoot but there is no evidence of abnormal function in the foot or toes when standing or when not bearing weight; voluntary actions are normal. In the course of review, the peculiar action is easily seen and the deformity which follows is quite obviously the result of this peculiar action; even so, the foot may still have a normal appearance at rest. If allowed to continue, the pes cavovarus previously observed only when walking, becomes fixed. The arch becomes higher, the forefoot more adducted and more inverted and the toes become clawed. This is usually unilateral and the result is not unlike the deformity seen in some late cases of poliomyelitis and cases of relapsed clubfoot (*Figure 4.1*).

Lower limbs

Examination of the lower limbs commonly reveals a shortening of one leg and foot although this is not always so. Discrepancy in limb length may increase to 2 inches, usually much less, but the shortening of the foot becomes exaggerated by the cavovarus and clawing of the toes. Peripheral circulatory deficiency is sometimes evident showing as lividity or cyanosis. In fully developed cases the combination of muscular imbalance and ischaemia produces fixed clawing with

26

atrophy of the toes although in some there is little actual clawing but considerable lateral deviation of all the outer toes, and hallux valgus.

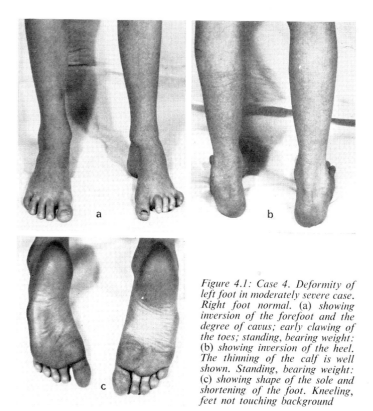

Figure 4.1: Case 4. Deformity of left foot in moderately severe case. Right foot normal. (a) showing inversion of the forefoot and the degree of cavus; early clawing of the toes; standing, bearing weight: (b) showing inversion of the heel. The thinning of the calf is well shown. Standing, bearing weight: (c) showing shape of the sole and shortening of the foot. Kneeling, feet not touching background

Nervous system

As in all progressive nervous conditions, the reflexes may be normal to begin with but change to exaggeration, diminution and finally vanish. Sensory changes are difficult to assess in children unless they are old enough to co-operate; even so their testimony cannot be relied on. We have had to rely on the more severe forms of sensory loss such as actual trophic ulceration, absence of plantar response or relatively symptomless fractures. Older children and adults are more easily assessed and may manifest the usual alterations in sensation in the leg of dulling of light touch, analgesia to pinprick, occasionally loss of postural sensibility and of vibration sense. The saddle area of the buttocks and also the anal reflex must always be tested.

Progression and later stages

Of our cases, 59 per cent presented because of the peculiarity of gait and foot deformity (which may be termed the orthopaedic syndrome), 26 per cent because of cutaneous manifestations on the back, 10 per cent because of bladder incontinence and the remaining 5 per cent because of scoliosis or foot trouble, for example, pain or ulceration.

In most cases the orthopaedic syndrome was well established before referral but a few cases came in the very early stages of deformity. Some already had altered reflexes while some lost reflexes during the preliminary review period or while waiting for admission to hospital; one developed spasticity of a lower limb during this period. While a number of children developed deformities and increased neurological deficit so that their abnormalities were comparable to those found in cases of spina bifida aperta, there was one change which carried a poor prognosis for recovery, namely when a cavovarus use of the foot resulting from overaction of the inverting muscles suddenly or within a short space of time altered to a paralytic valgus.

The adults all came to us late, some with incontinence of a few years' duration and some with established foot deformities (since childhood) and sensory loss; 2 had trophic ulceration. One was the case, cited earlier, who had no neurological deficit or muscle imbalance but had a hypersensitive naevoid patch on her back, and hypertrichosis.

REFERENCES

James, C. C. M. and Lassman, L. P. (1960). 'Spinal Dysraphism. An Orthopaedic Syndrome in Children Accompanying Occult Forms.' *Archs. Dis. Childh.* **35**, 315
— — (1962a). 'Spinal Dysraphism. The Diagnosis and Treatment of Progressive Lesions in Spina Bifida Occulta.' *J. Bone Jt. Surg.* **44B**, 828
— — (1962b). 'Spinal Dysraphism. Spinal Cord Lesions Associated with Spina Bifida Occulta.' *Physiotherapy* **48**, 154

5—Radiology

Radiology consists of three separate investigations, namely survey radiography, tomography and myelography.

SURVEY RADIOGRAPHY

The whole spine is recorded from the occipito-atlantoid joint to the tip of the coccyx. The principal purposes are to determine the existence and extent of congenital laminal anomalies, increase of interpedicular distance, congenital vertebral body abnormalities, narrowing of intervertebral disc spaces and the presence of the bone septa associated with diastematomyelia.

Laminal anomalies

In every case in this series there was a laminal defect at one or more levels from Cv7 to Sv5. No anomalies were detected in Cv1 to 6. Table 5.1 shows the levels most commonly affected; 7 cases have been omitted, 3 because they were too young to make an accurate diagnosis, 3 because their radiographs are no longer available and information is incomplete, and 1 case (15) where there was sacral somatoschisis. It will be seen that deficiencies of the laminae of Lv5 constituted 18 per cent of all laminal defects but these occurred in 82 cases. Similarly, 16 per cent of all laminal deficiencies occurred at Sv1 level and were found in 73 cases. Abnormality of both Lv5 and Sv1 laminae was seen in 66 cases. While in the majority of cases, defects were localized over 3 or 4 pairs of laminae, a few had very extensive anomalies, for example, Tv11–Sv5. Anomalies in the lower thoracic spine were accompanied by laminal defects in the lumbar region. In 5 cases there were 6 lumbar vertebrae present, in one case there were 4 lumbar vertebrae and 13 thoracic and in 2 cases there were 4 lumbar vertebrae.

In our criteria for undertaking laminectomy, we stipulate that laminal defects should be greater than a simple split of the spinous process of Sv1. In this series, 3 cases had a defect of only these laminae and in 1 of them there were also increased inter-pedicular distances at Lv4–Sv2. Clinical considerations necessitated

TABLE 5.1

DISTRIBUTION OF LAMINAL DEFECTS

(*percentage frequency in 93 cases*)

Cervical and thoracic spine		
Tv9–12 (all equally)	7	
Other levels	3	10
Lumbar spine		
Lv1	3	
Lv2	7	
Lv3	9	
Lv4	13	
Lv5	18	50
Sacrum		
Sv1	16	
Sv2	10	
Sv3	7	
Sv4	4	
Sv5	3	40
		100

further investigation of these cases and myelography showed ab-normality in 2. The third case (74) had a normal myelogram and the conus was at Lv2/3 level; at operation the only abnormality was a tight filum terminale (p. 84). A defect of Lv5 laminae alone occurred in only 1 case (99) and this was associated with pedicular erosion; an intramedullary dermoid cyst was found at operation.

Increased interpedicular distance

The distance between the pedicles was measurably increased in 79 cases. In the remaining 21 cases the fact of normal interpedicular distance was recorded in 18 and in 6 of these the absence of increased widening is unexpected; 5 had diastematomyelia (4 without septum) and one had an intramedullary dermoid cyst (without flattening of the pedicles). These 6 cases contrast with the other 36 cases of diastematomyelia and 2 other cases of intramedullary dermoid cyst in the whole series.

Of the 12 other cases without increased widening, no intrathecal abnormality was detected at operation in 2, 1 had a lipoma in the terminal theca and 6 had forms of meningocele manqué with adhesions and bands relating to the cauda equina (5 cases) or the terminal spinal cord. The remaining 3 cases had a subcutaneous lumbosacral lipoma directly continuous intrathecally with the filum terminale (2 cases) or the terminal spinal cord.

Flattening of the pedicles was seen on radiography in only 2 cases each with a dermoid cyst, 1 intramedullary within the conus medullaris and 1 with multiple adhesions amongst the distal cauda equina.

Abnormalities of vertebral bodies, sacrum and intervertebral discs

Abnormalities of the centra were detected in 20 cases. Five had thoracic hemivertebrae (including Case 72, *see below*), 1 had a vertical cleft of Tv11 with a portion of the body developed with each pedicle (Case 60) and 6 had small centra—thoracic, lumbar or sacral; 5 cases had a narrowed anteroposterior diameter of lumbar vertebral bodies, 2 of which also had associated widening of the transverse diameter. In 3 cases there was fusion of adjacent vertebral bodies, from Tv9 to Lv2 (Case 34), of Cv2/3 (Case 67) and of Tv3/4 together with Tv5/6 (Case 81).

Congenital narrowing of intervertebral discs was noted in 17 cases, 7 of them associated with diastematomyelia at the same level (6 with a septum, 1 without) and 3 in cases with diastematomyelia at an unassociated different level (1 with septum, 2 without). The remaining 7 cases were associated with various forms of meningocele manqué.

In 1 case there was bifid development of the sacrum (Case 15) while in 6 other cases there was agenesis of the sacrum relating to the terminal sacral segments—Sv3–5 in Cases 34, 60 and 67, and Sv4–5 in Cases 7, 8 and 72.

Spondylolisthesis at Lv5/Sv1 was found in 1 case.

Bone septa

Bone septa were detected in 16 cases on survey radiography. At laminectomy these were all confirmed and one other case was found where the septum was partially ossified.

TOMOGRAPHY

After examination of 19 cases by tomography, this investigation has not been carried out since Case 57 because it has proved to be unnecessary and exposes the individual to excessive radiation.

Originally, tomography was intended to define the existence and size of a septum in diastematomyelia and the shape and nature of laminal abnormalities, particularly inversion. Our experience suggests that tomography is an academic exercise in spinal dysraphism because the same information can be obtained from myelography.

MYELOGRAPHY

Myelography is performed to demonstrate abnormalities of the flow of the radiopaque medium, space-occupying lesions and filling defects. It is also used to detect the level of the conus medullaris, the course of the anterior spinal artery, the width of the filum terminale and the termination of the dural sac (*Figure 5.1*). With few exceptions, the examinations in this series were carried out by Dr. G. L. Gryspeerdt, using the technique he originated and has described (1963), most particularly, examination of the patient in the supine position which is essential to diagnosis in spinal dysraphism.

Myodil (Pantopaque) is introduced by the cisternal route using general anaesthesia in children. Earlier, the lumbar route was used but, since the conus medullaris is often at a very low level in spinal dysraphism, we considered that this route was possibly more dangerous; also, failure to inject all the contrast medium into the subarachnoid space obscures the detail in an important area and the extra-arachnoid material remains unabsorbed for several weeks so that subsequent screening has to be postponed unduly. With cisternal myelography, there is always the risk of encountering a case with an Arnold–Chiari malformation but examination of the survey radiographs and the patient's clinical abnormality will usually give warning of the likelihood of its presence. The Arnold–Chiari malformation has not been found by supine myelography in any of our cases of occult spinal dysraphism and is likely to be encountered only if a myelomeningocele with good skin cover is mistaken for a lumbosacral lipoma (Chapter 15). In later cases after this series, when the malformation has been suspected, we have either introduced the Myodil into a lateral ventricle or by the lumbar route.

Reaction to Myodil in this series occurred in 2 out of 24 cases after lumbar route injection; both suffered from some neck stiffness and vomiting. Similarly, 4 out of 76 cases injected by the cisternal route were affected; 3 suffered from neck stiffness, headache and moderate pyrexia, the fourth case was drowsy for 2 days with high pyrexia but without neck stiffness. After either of these procedures a few cases were mildly pyrexial but in most the cause was ascribed to infection of the upper respiratory or urinary tracts.

Findings at myelography

In only 8 cases was no abnormality found at myelography. Of these, 2 were early cases in which the conus medullaris was not identified; in neither case was there an intrathecal abnormality found at opera-

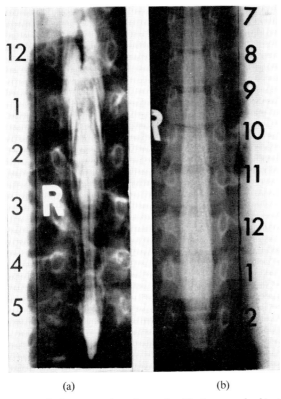

(a)   (b)

Figure 5.1. Demonstration of conus level in the normal subject. (a) Supine examination; the filum terminale is of normal calibre and widens out into the conus at the Lv1/Lv2 level. (b) Prone examination: the anterior spinal artery can be traced downwards through the thoracic region to the level of Lv1 but no lower. The great anterior radicular artery enters the anterior spinal artery from the left side at Tv11 level

tion. Of the other 6 cases, 3 had a meningocele manqué, 1 a dermal sinus connecting with the conus medullaris, 1 had myodysplasia and 1 had a lumbosacral lipoma connecting to the filum terminale.

In all the remaining cases in this series, there were filling defects,

33

space-occupying lesions, translucencies associated with fibrous bands, aberrant nerve roots or a septum, a block to the flow of Myodil, an abnormally low-placed conus medullaris or an abnormally wide filum terminale. These last 2 items require further discussion.

Low-placed conus medullaris and increased width of the filum terminale

These 2 factors are of diagnostic importance. They are demonstrated by myelography in the supine position although the anterior spinal artery as seen in prone myelography will often give an indication that the conus medullaris is situated abnormally low without giving its exact location.

Supine examinations started with Case 3 in this series but the technique for identification of the situation of the terminal spinal cord was not worked out for some time although subsequent review shows that accurate location was quickly achieved. The conus medullaris was not looked for in Cases 1–4, it was not defined in Cases 7, 11 and 12 and 6 other subsequent cases in these series, in most of which the conus medullaris was found at operation to be at the normal level. When the conus medullaris is at the normal level it is often very difficult to demarcate and we have regarded the normal level as being cranial to the cranial border of Lv3 body. While it is known that the conus medullaris lies over the body of Lv3 in a small percentage of normal people, we have always regarded this level as on the borderline of abnormality and taking other radiographic and clinical features into consideration have operated on a number of cases. In only 6 cases in this series were the myelograms completely normal with the conus medullaris identified as lying at Lv2, Lv2/3 disc, or Lv3 (p. 33); in all of them at subsequent operation an abnormality was found which required treatment and the location of the spinal cord was confirmed. In all other cases with a normal level of the conus medullaris, the myelogram showed some other abnormality.

Location of the conus medullaris by myelography in this series has been accurate as confirmed by operation, an error of one segment is negligible and could be due to miscounting by the surgeon who is very much concerned with the detail of what is often a very difficult operation. In only 3 cases was the myelographic identification in error by more than one segment but this made no difficulty for the surgeon who had other indications as to the area to be explored.

The key to identification of the conus medullaris by myelography in the supine position is the demonstration of the filum terminale, a structure which normally measures less than 2 mm in diameter on the radiograph. A width of 2 mm raises suspicion of abnormality while 3 mm or more is definitely abnormal. Some cases showing an apparent widening of the cranial part of the filum terminale at myelography were found at operation to have an attenuated conus medullaris, accounting for the appearance. In 18 cases (including Cases 1 and 2) the filum terminale was not identified, in 39 cases it was regarded as normal and in 43 cases it was widened (including 4 cases where the conus medullaris was not detected).

At operation, widening of the filum terminale in most cases is seen to result from adherence of the terminal nerves of the cauda equina, but in a few it is an intrinsic thickening and is associated with adhesions to the dura mater. It has not been found to be associated with any particular syndrome or with any particular spinal cord abnormality but it happens that we have had to operate on every case where the filum terminale was shown to be wider than normal at myelography and have always found some intrathecal abnormality.

The myelogram showed no abnormality except a low-placed conus medullaris in 10 cases. In a further 7 cases the only abnormality was a low-placed conus medullaris and a widened filum terminale. Survey radiography of these cases indicated an increased inter-pedicular distance in all but 3. In each of these 17 cases an abnormality was found at operation in the lower lumbar or sacral region, 11 of them having some form of meningocele manqué. Nevertheless, examination of the association of level of conus medullaris and widening of the filum terminale with the type and site of abnormality found at operation shows no correlation. A widened filum terminale is not associated with any particular level of the conus medullaris nor the proximity to it of the spinal cord abnormality.

REFERENCE

Gryspeerdt, G. L. (1963). 'Myelographic Assessment of Occult Forms of Spinal Dysraphism.' *Acta radiol.* **1**, 702

6—Diagnosis and Treatment

The very early case is not easy to diagnose and the progress of deterioration may have to be watched over a period. Survey radiography of the spine will show laminal defects of a greater degree than a simple split in the spinous process of Sv1 (Chapter 5) and myelography will demonstrate a major abnormality or a low situated conus medullaris (Chapter 5). When those two radiological examinations are positive the diagnosis becomes established. Our experience and morbid anatomical studies suggest that in the absence of greater degrees of laminal defect, a surgically treatable abnormality of the spinal cord and nerve roots is unlikely to be present.

In the first place, the diagnosis depends upon the presenting symptoms. Pain is unusual but, if present, may suggest a march fracture, osteochondritis of a metatarsal head, foot-strain or lumbar nerve root irritation. The peculiar gait suggests many conditions, a verruca, early hallux rigidus, injury to the sesamoids underlying the first metatarsal head, too small a shoe or early pes cavus presenting in one foot.

The cases of short foot and leg of the variety so common in orthopaedic practice and for which no cause is found are distinguishable from those due to spinal dysraphism because there is no change in foot function or deformity and no neurological deficit in the course of prolonged review; a personal series of such cases showed a very high incidence of minimal spina bifida on radiography. Other possible causes of leg and foot discrepancy are old bone infection, previous fracture, hemihypertrophy and angiomatosis.

In our experience, the principal conditions needing to be excluded are cerebral palsy, usually in the form of mild hemiplegia, Friedreich's ataxia and old poliomyelitis. It is important not to accept this last diagnosis or a history of old injury without very careful enquiry: both these diagnoses are commonly applied *post hoc* to account for foot deformity of obscure origin.

Other diseases of the nervous system to be considered in the differential diagnosis are spinal cord tumours, neurofibromatosis and all those mentioned by Brewerton, Sandifer and Sweetman (1963) and Heron (1969) in their investigations of pes cavus, including peroneal muscular atrophy, polyneuritis, Roussy–Levy syndrome and the hereditary cerebellar ataxia of Marie.

In the long term, the limb deformity and the neurological deficit, particularly incontinence, make the diagnosis straightforward.

The treatment of the primary cause is exploration of the affected area of the spinal cord or cauda equina indicated by myelography, for example, the low conus medullaris in the absence of any other abnormality. Consideration of the age and frailty of the patient, the duration of the symptoms and the severity of the deficit may satisfy the surgeon that the condition has existed too long to benefit by major surgery so that only local ameliorative procedures are justified. Recently a man aged 66 years with a 2-year history of neurogenic incontinence did not benefit from surgical exploration, but a woman aged 44 years (Case 95) recovered power in one leg which had become progressively weaker over a period of about 10 years although her incontinence, present for 6 years, was unaltered. A man aged 19 years (Case 75) with lower limb symptoms and incontinence from early childhood was improved.

REFERENCES

Brewerton, D. A., Sandifer, P. H. and Sweetman, D. R. (1963). '"Ideopathic" Pes Cavus. An Investigation into its Aetiology.' *Br. med. J.* **2**, 659

Heron, J. R. (1969). 'Neurological Syndromes Associated with Pes Cavus.' *Proc. R. Soc. Med.* **62**, 270

7—Anaesthesia

J. D. Whitby

General anaesthesia is required for two procedures in the management of cases of spinal dysraphism in children. The first is cisternal
myelography. This takes place mainly in the dark, or in subdued
lighting if an image intensifier is being used, and necessitates considerable tilting of the patient into both head-up and head-down
positions. The second is laminectomy.

Premedication for myelography
Premedication is largely a matter of individual preference. Intramuscular atropine, 0·15–0·4 mg depending upon the age, has been
given in all cases. Intramuscular droperidol in doses of approximately 0·1 mg/kg, given one hour before induction, has been used in
many cases, and an opiate or pethidine for some of the older children, but when the child has been between the ages of 1 and 7 years,
he has usually been given full basal sedation.

At first this was achieved with rectal thiopentone. Recently we
have been using a 10 per cent solution of methohexitone in water. A
dose of 10 mg/lb (2·2 mg/kg) is given 25 to 30 minutes before the
induction proper. The difference between the two drugs when given
rectally is similar to that seen when they are given intravenously and
the timing is more critical with the shorter acting methohexitone than
with the thiopentone.

In these cases the atropine is given 5 to 10 minutes after the
methohexitone when the child is asleep. This means that the time
allowed for it to act is less than usual. Consequently the respiratory
passages may be a little moist during the early stages of anaesthesia,
but the amount of secretion is small and it is easily removed by
suction. Giving the atropine after the methohexitone avoids an
injection while the child is conscious. For the same reason, specimens
of blood for haemoglobin estimation, grouping and cross-matching
are taken after the child has been anaesthetized.

Some form of napkin to avoid soiling is advisable when rectal premedication has been used, but the use of safety pins is not permissible. A square of Gamgee fastened anterolaterally with adhesive plaster has proved satisfactory.

Anaesthesia

Inflammable and explosive gases can not be used in a radiography department, so nitrous oxide, halothane and trichloroethylene are the inhalation agents of choice. Intravenous barbiturates are optional for induction, depending upon the age of the child and the premedication used. Intubation is necessary and the relaxation required for this has been achieved with either suxamethonium or halothane. Spontaneous respiration is preferable to controlled respiration, which is unnecessary and would only complicate the management of anaesthesia in the dark. An open T-piece circuit with a small-bore tube for fresh gases is more convenient for maintenance than a semi-closed one with wide-bore corrugated tubing, even in older children.

Cisternal puncture

An increase in cerebrospinal fluid pressure will facilitate cisternal puncture. Searching for a collapsed cistern is both difficult and dangerous. Therefore the usual considerations governing the administration of a neurosurgical anaesthetic can and should be ignored. The marked flexion of the head and spine in the lateral position required for the puncture tends to raise the cerebrospinal fluid pressure, but digital pressure exerted on the jugular vein by the anaesthetist is also helpful. If under these conditions the cerebrospinal fluid does not spurt out when the cistern is entered, it is probable that the bevel of the needle is only partly in the subarachnoid space and that any attempt to inject the Myodil at this stage will result in part of the medium passing into the subdural or extradural spaces.

Complications

The complications encountered so far that have been severe enough to cause a postponement of the examination have been as follows.

(1) Apnoea of several minutes' duration, with or without an associated cardiac arrhythmia, following insertion of the needle.

(2) Apnoea on turning a child prone after a very heavily blood-stained aspiration of cerebrospinal fluid.

(3) The repeated aspiration of pure blood or very heavily blood-stained cerebrospinal fluid.

(4) Extra-arachnoid injection of the Myodil.

Slight bloodstaining of the aspirated cerebrospinal fluid can be ignored, although it may cause some postoperative discomfort.

Myelography

As soon as the Myodil has been injected, the table is given a 5-degree head-up tilt to prevent the medium from running up into the basal

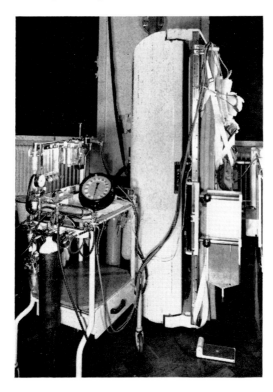

Figure 7.1. Myelogram table with maximum head-up elevation, showing the anaesthetic machine, pulsometer-sphygmomanometer and the combined anaesthetic and monitoring leads attached to the head of the table

cisterns. Care must be taken to keep the child parallel with the table and his head extended while turning him over into the prone position for the first part of the examination, in order to prevent the Myodil from leaving the cervical region in either direction.

The maximum inclination employed in either direction is usually between 40 and 60 degrees from the horizontal plane. Occasionally it may be necessary to tilt the patient up to 80 degrees, or even vertically, in order to examine the upper cervical region for an Arnold–Chiari malformation, to return the Myodil down into the terminal theca, or to ⌐drain the myodil out of a meningocele (*Figure 7.1*). When the child is supine, the Myodil can usually be drained out of the fourth ventricle and the cisterna magna with only moderate tilting, by raising the head off the table. Fortunately the blood pressure of a child tends to be more resistant to changes of

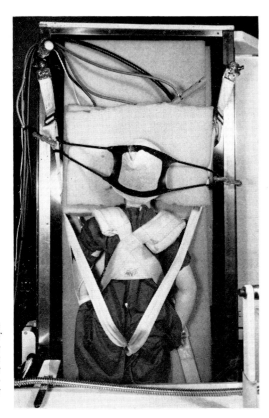

Figure 7.2. Child prone for the first stage of myelography, showing the harness for the trunk and the Connell harness and shock cord for restraining the head during extreme tilting

posture under anaesthesia than that of an adult. Also there is no question of any diminished circulatory volume due to blood or fluid loss and the more extreme tilts do not have to be maintained for more than a minute or two at a time. We have not encountered any severe falls of blood pressure so far.

For these reasons firm fixation to the table is essential. The child lies on a polyfoam mattress. The head rests in a semicircular depression cut in two squares of polyfoam and is prevented from

41

falling backwards in the prone position and forwards in the supine position by a bandage or by a Connell anaesthetic harness attached to the sides of the table with shock cord. The trunk is fastened to the table by a harness of parachute webbing. The straps should be tight enough to prevent the body from slipping when tilted, but not so tight as to impede the ventilatory excursion. A bandage is also fixed across the legs just above the ankles. The arms are by the side (*Figure 7.2*).

When the child is turned over into the supine position, the wrists are joined by a bandage and the surplus ends are led up to the head

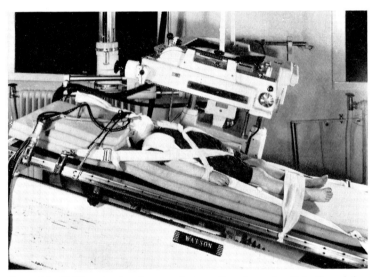

Figure 7.3. Child supine for the second stage of myelography. Note the polyfoam pads with semicircular cut-outs into which the head fits, the restraining bandage across the ankles, the bandage for raising the arms in order to take a lateral view, and the attachment of all anaesthetic and monitoring leads to a short upright pillar at the head of the table

of the table. This allows the anaesthetist to raise the child's arms above its head when the radiologist wishes to take a lateral view (*Figure 7.3*).

Monitoring during myelography

Both respiration and heartbeat should be carefully monitored during all stages of the investigation. This can be done simply by using a stethoscope with long tubing. One limb is attached to a plastic chest piece fastened on to the precordium. A well stretched rubber diaphragm made out of the finger of a surgical glove will improve its acoustic qualities. The other limb is attached to the side-arm of a second Ayre's T-piece which is inserted into the exhaust tubing of the open respiratory circuit. Some anaesthetists may prefer to use a plastic oesophageal stethoscope instead of the precordial chest piece.

Monitoring the blood pressure in the dark is more difficult. The main problem is to achieve a satisfactory illumination of the sphygmo-manometer dial without interfering with the dark-adaption of the radiologist. Luminous paint is inadequate as both figures and pointer are too small to show up clearly, even when a large dial is used. However, with the 7-inch Accosan model it is possible to replace the metal face with a partially blacked-out transparent Perspex one and to illuminate both scale and pointer from behind. There is also room to build a pulsometer into the casing, the batteries being mounted in a box on the back to allow easy replacement. The pulsometer used in this unit has a red winking light signal and also gives out an audible tick. The intensity of the light signal is con-trolled by a rheostat.

The sphygmomanometer dial was originally illuminated by three 2·5 volt torch bulbs mounted in series, the intensity again being controlled by a rheostat. The disadvantages of this method were the unevenness of the illumination, the drain on the pulsometer battery and the fact that the failure of one bulb or its connections meant the failure of all three.

Our present model uses two semicircular Betalights mounted behind the dial. These produce a very satisfactory illumination under all lighting conditions and have a half-life of between ten and twenty years.* An additional small Betalight provided for mounting on the pointer has proved unnecessary.

It is convenient to use different colours of rubber for the various tubes leading to and from the patient so that their function can be easily distinguished, and to form them into a single cord by encircling all the components with rubber bands at 12-inch intervals.

This combined cord, which is kept as a special set for myelography, is strapped to a short upright pillar at the upper and outer end of the table (*Figure 7.3*). The tubing must be long enough to allow for the rise and fall of the head of the table. To avoid having to use an unmanageable length of tubing, the horizontal movement which also occurs during tilting is best covered by moving the anaesthetic machine along the side of the table.

* Obtainable from Saunders-Roe Nuclear Enterprises Ltd.

Laminectomy

The premedication and induction of anaesthesia are the same as for the myelography. After the induction an intravenous cannula is inserted percutaneously, preferably into a vein on the dorsum of the hand, and a dextrose-saline drip started.

It is essential that the position of the patient during laminectomy should be one which will not in any way impede full respiratory movement. The abdomen must be clear of the underlying table during inspiration as well as expiration, to prevent any increase in intra-abdominal pressure and congestion of the extradural venous plexus. It is also desirable to flatten out the lumbosacral curve. To achieve this, we use the prone position with the thighs well flexed, the anterior superior iliac spines being supported on sandbags and the chest on polyfoam pads.

Even when the position is perfect in these respects, the surgical dissection in cases with lipomata or tracts leading down to the dura from the skin will not keep to the anatomical tissue planes and more bleeding must be expected than would be the case in a laminectomy for a prolapsed lumbar intervertebral disc in an adult. Blood loss varies more with the nature of the lesion than with the age of the child, but the smaller the child, the greater any given blood loss will be in proportion to its total blood volume. We have transfused these cases routinely, although occasionally the indication has been marginal, making due allowance for postoperative as well as operative blood loss.

Although we have used controlled hyperventilation in a number of cases, it has not had any obvious effect on the total operative blood loss, whether judged visually from the swabs, drapes and contents of the suction bottle or estimated from them by an extraction and calorimetric method.

If controlled ventilation is used, care must be taken to ensure that the tidal volume is not so large that it forces the abdomen against the table with each inflation, thus increasing intra-abdominal pressure and causing venous congestion. This error may have been the cause of the tidal wave of cerebrospinal fluid that flooded the operating area with each inspiration in the first case in which we used artificial ventilation. With the smaller child in particular, any ventilator used must allow the tidal volume to be measured accurately because with the patient prone, covered up by towels and surrounded by the surgical team, it is impossible to see or judge the amount of thoracic or abdominal movement.

With children under an age of 1 year, a warm water bed is used to prevent heat loss as the normal working temperature of the

44

theatre in this unit is between 18 and 21°C. With older children Gamgee and polythene covering is sufficient. Either the pharyngeal or the lower oesophageal temperature is monitored.

Postoperative course

The postoperative course after laminectomy is a painful one and the children lie still and are reluctant to move for the first 2 days. Adequate analgesia during this period is essential (Chapter 9). The improvement on the third day is often striking.

8—Principles of Surgery

The only method of treatment is surgical removal of extrinsic abnormalities likely to fix the spinal cord in its position so that it cannot move or which cause pressure upon the nervous tissue. Occasionally, owing to adhesions or interspersal of fat and fibrous tissue among nerve roots, it is only possible to leave the area decompressed as will naturally follow the laminectomy, provided the dura mater is not closed too tightly.

Basically the operation consists in retracting the muscles to expose the laminae, removing the required number of laminae and spinous processes and opening the dura mater so that the spinal cord and nerve roots can be clearly seen. Usually a minimum or 3 pairs of laminae must be taken away so that the dura may be opened where the underlying structures are likely to be normal. It is essential to have an exposure as wide as this so that the spinal cord can be properly inspected; it may be necessary to remove 4 or 5 pairs of laminae in order to complete the operation in a small child but the less bone removed, the less likely is the vertebral column to be weakened. The interarticular joints are not interfered with so that the spine continues to function well. The risk of developing scoliosis subsequently is slight; in our series the only case to require subsequent spinal fusion for this reason already had scoliosis as a result of hemivertebrae and similar bone anomalies and the spinal curvature became rapidly worse after laminectomy. Following this case the operations in the presence of existing scoliosis have been of very limited scope which makes for considerable technical difficulties and possibly incomplete exploration.

The site of laminectomy is usually indicated by the myelography findings. It is necessary to locate the abnormality in relation to the vertebral body level and to decide whether this site should be approached through the laminae cranial or caudal; all 3 pairs of laminae will have to be removed in any case and the site of abnormality should

46

never be approached directly. Where the only myelographic abnormality is a low-placed conus, it is usually approached through the laminae immediately cranial to the conus and the exploration continued in a caudal direction. When the myelogram has shown 2 abnormalities widely apart, the more caudal one should be operated on first, leaving the cranial one and keeping the patient under review in case a second operation should become necessary. A longitudinal midline incision is used and this can be elongated to obtain a wider exposure if necessary.

In some cases there is a positive indication on the skin surface for the placing of the incision. A lipoma has to be circumscribed and undercut so as to detect its deep continuation or pedicle (*see Figure 15.4*) which is then followed to its point of entry into the neural arch, and the laminae cranial to this point will need to be removed; the myelogram will have given an indication of where this pedicle attaches, usually in the region of the conus, and this continuation of the lipoma pedicle may well pass cranially extradurally and intradurally as many as 3 neural arches. Similarly, with a fistula or sinus its track must be dissected out and kept in continuity until its ultimate point of attachment is located. Occasionally a dermal sinus or dimple is situated at a considerable distance from the abnormality shown on the myelogram, in which case it can be ignored in the initial incision provided it is certain that it is not fistulous; if the exploration within the theca indicates that there is a deep connection from the sinus, it can be cut off its deep attachment and followed from within just as far as necessary to make sure it can no longer affect the intrathecal structures. If it turns out to be fistulous, the dissection must be extensive so that the whole track is excised. In exactly the same way, a scarred area on the skin surface as of a healed meningocele must be circumscribed and its deep attachment followed.

The other forms of cutaneous abnormality can be ignored unless in a case of hypertrichosis the area of origin is small; it is then kindest to the patient to excise the hair-bearing skin and close the skin defect by a direct suture, but it is rare for the origin of the hypertrichosis to be so circumscribed.

Except in the types of case already mentioned, there is not usually any detectable band or connection from the skin and muscles down to the bone so that exposure of the neural arches is straightforward. Where the laminae are defective, the gaps are filled with fibrous tissue with an admixture of fat sometimes of considerable extent. It is common for one or more bands to connect from the deep surface of this material to the dura, or from the interspinous spaces (or from the joints between the neural arches) and these may not be

47

detected until they are found lying loose on the dura mater after the laminae have been removed. They attach to the dura mater at a more cranial level and usually in the midline.

With the removal of the laminae, the dura mater is exposed and it will be clear whether there are two dural tubes as occurs with diastematomyelia associated with a septum or whether there are extradural bands present. If there is a septum passing between two dural tubes, it is best removed at this point as the dura mater assists in preventing damage to neural tissue during the manipulations of instruments in the process and the gap between the two tubes may be very small or the septum very close fitting. The dura mater surrounding the septum is gently separated from it by blunt dissection and with a Pennybacker's rongeur the spur is removed piecemeal until its base has been made flush with the anterior wall of the spinal canal. It may be impossible to excise the spur completely at this stage and the remainder may have to be removed when the dura mater has been opened: in some cases where the gap posteriorly through the cord is not big enough to allow removal of the vertebral end of the bone septum the spinal cord must be elevated by cutting one of the ligamenta denticulata and using this to rotate it so that the remainder of the spur can be excised anteriorly to the spinal cord. There is always some haemorrhage from the deep attachment of the septum to the vertebral body and this commonly ceases once the base of the septum is completely removed but occasionally the area has to be cauterized when the gap between the two dural tubes is too small for wax to be pressed in.

The dura mater is opened in the midline usually cranial to the point of attachment of an extradural band or pedicle from the subcutaneous tissues, but occasionally there are indications for starting caudal to this. It must be remembered that in the embryo these bands probably passed vertically internally but with growth of the body and movement of the spinal cord in a cranial direction, the bands are likely to take an oblique course to end at a more cranial level than their point of dural attachment and even more cranial than their subcutaneous origin. This being so, the dural incision must start well away so that as the edges of the dura mater are retracted, the intrathecal contents can be clearly seen and bands and nervous tissue can be left unharmed. Where there are two dural tubes, each must be opened in the midline so that ultimately the intermediate dura mater can be freed from internal structures and entirely removed. If this intermediate dura mater is not removed, it will continue to act as a septum liable to press on the neural tissue and be a continuing preventive of spinal cord mobility.

48

The whole of the intrathecal structures are now available for inspection and the myelogram may well have given an indication what abnormality is to be expected. The intrathecal continuation of an extradural band is sometimes very difficult to locate because it may be fine and adherent to the internal surface of the dura mater and concealed by a fold in the dura mater. These intrathecal bands may occasionally loop in a caudal direction rather than with the more usual cranial obliquity from the point of penetration of the dura mater but they continue to become attached to the spinal cord, or to bands passing between the two spinal cords of a diastemato-myelia; they must be cut from their attachment so as to release any traction effect and this is safe to do as they no longer have any function since their extradural continuation has already been severed. Microscopy shows them to be either posterior nerve roots or dense fibrous strands, presumably posterior roots which have atrophied owing to absence of function as a result of ectopia of the neural crest cells (*see* Table 2.1). Care must be taken to make sure that the intrathecal portion is not merely a strand holding a loop of nerves up to the dura mater. The strand can be divided to release the loop from its adherence to the dura mater. The loop consists of nerve roots or tracts which emerge from the spinal cord or cauda equina and then return to near their point of origin; we believe that this looping of nerves is an indication that at this point a meningocele was almost formed so that for convenience we classify this type of abnormality as a meningocele manqué (Chapter 14). This finding in the theca is frequently associated with the scarred area of the skin which resembles an atrophied meningocele and is also found in those children whose meningoceles present at birth have fibrosed down and healed over.

The most difficult abnormalities to deal with are those where there is fat and fibrous tissue between the nerves of the cauda equina and those where the dura mater is adherent to the dorsal surface of the spinal cord. With the former it may not be possible to free the nerve roots completely and the surgeon has to be satisfied that by removing the laminae he has at least decompressed the area. This problem is avoided in cases of lumbosacral lipoma by turning the lipoma cranially so that its pedicle is pulled away from the region of the terminal dural sac and in so doing frees itself from the cauda equina. The pedicle then presents its ventral surface and its attach-ment to the spinal cord is easily seen. The pedicle is cut off the spinal cord at this point. The adherence of the dura mater to the dorsum of the spinal cord can sometimes be freed by blunt dissection provided that the exposure gives clear vision and that it can be seen that the nerve roots are not also adherent. If the nerve roots are adherent, there is usually insufficient visibility and the dura mater has to be left untouched.

Having dealt with the abnormality affecting the nervous tissue, the subarachnoid space under the untouched laminae must be inspected both cranially and caudally to ensure that there are no further bands, adhesions or other abnormalities and that there is no longer any tissue left which will interfere with movement of the spinal cord nor exert pressure on it or the nerve roots.

The filum terminale is normally a fine structure with a blood vessel running on its dorsal surface but occasionally it is widened owing to adherence of nerve roots running alongside it. After the dura mater has been opened and the cerebrospinal fluid has escaped the filum terminale falls back against the vertebral bodies; if it does not do so it is either being held away by adhesions or is tight. The adhesions must be freed to release it or it must be divided as far caudally as possible after freeing any adherent nerve roots. A filum terminale which is not tight separates its cut ends by about 0·5 cm if the division is made near the termination of the dural sac but this distance will be increased if the cut is made near the lumbosacral joint because the weight of the spinal cord pulls it down the incline of the lumbar lordosis. The operating table should be tilted to obviate this gravity effect before cutting the filum terminale and gaps measuring 1·0 to 2·5 cm have been obtained in cases where the filum had previously been strung up like a bow-string.

The operation having been completed, the dura mater is sutured with 0000 Mersilene on 20-mm half-circle eyeless round-bodied needles to make a watertight closure. In some cases at the end of the operation a dural defect which cannot be closed by suture is present and this must be grafted by fascia from the posterior layer of the lumbar aponeurosis or from the fascia lata on the outer side of the thigh; the muscles are then closed with 0 Mersilene on No. 10 half-circle triangular-pointed needles. The skin and subcutaneous tissues are closed in two layers, the deeper layer with 000 Mersilene sutures on 22 mm spring-eye round-bodied needles and the skin with the same suture material on No. 13 half-circle triangular-pointed needles. A firm pressure dressing is applied to the wound and when this is low it is sealed off from the anus by the application of water-proof plastic adhesive tape to the lower part of the dressing.

9—Postoperative Care and Complications

POSTOPERATIVE CARE

The child is nursed on the side and the position changed 2-hourly or more frequently if desired; the pressure areas are treated 4-hourly. The temperature, pulse, respiration and blood pressure are all recorded. Half-hourly pulse and 2-hourly temperature checks are continued for at least 12 hours, and then the blood pressure is recorded only when required. Adequate postoperative sedation must be maintained, and pethidine is given intramuscularly every 6–8 hours for the first 36–48 hours. Intravenous therapy is continued with 4·3 per cent dextrose and 0·18 per cent saline, following the blood transfusion which is begun immediately the patient is anaesthetized and before the operation is started. Intake and output of fluids must be strictly recorded. Routine postoperative antibiotic therapy is not prescribed. If retention of urine with overflow occurs the bladder is expressed manually every 3–4 hours, or a Gibbons catheter is introduced into the bladder and continuous drainage maintained until normal function is resumed. The intravenous therapy is discontinued after 12–16 hours, provided the child is taking fluids and not vomiting.

On the third postoperative day movement is encouraged, and an aperient is given if necessary. On the fourth postoperative day the patient is provided with extra pillows, and then encouraged to sit up and play.

The dressing should be left untouched until the seventh day unless the patient develops pyrexia or the dressing becomes contaminated with cerebrospinal fluid. On the seventh day the wound is inspected and re-dressed.

The patient is allowed up for bed-making and watching television on the seventh postoperative day if satisfactory progress is being maintained. On the eighth day alternate sutures are removed from

51

the wound and check radiographs of the spine are taken. The patient is allowed to stand and walk.

On the tenth postoperative day the remaining sutures are removed, and by this time the patient should be ambulant. The following day the patient is discharged home, to be followed up at frequent intervals in the out-patient department.

TABLE 9.1

POSTOPERATIVE COURSE AND COMPLICATIONS

No complications	81
Acute dilatation of the stomach	1
Serious postoperative shock	1
Wound infection—early	5
—delayed	1
Cerebrospinal fluid fistula	11
100 Cases: Mortality—Nil	

Urinary retention of short duration occurs after almost all the operations and is regarded as normal.

Acute dilatation of the stomach

The single case of acute dilatation was of some interest because it occurred in a boy aged 4 years 4 months on whom we operated at another hospital away from our own unit. The dilatation rapidly responded to continuous aspiration of the stomach and intravenous therapy: we are unable to account for its occurrence unless it can be regarded as a shock response to release of tension on the spinal cord. At operation the filum terminale and nerve roots of the left cauda equina were found to be adherent to the dura mater dorsally (a form of meningocele manqué). The adhesions were divided and the tight filum terminale was cut leaving a gap of 2·75 cm. Prior to operation he had had diurnal enuresis and instead of developing retention postoperatively as do most cases, he had frequency of micturition which steadily subsided. Three and a half years later he had good bladder control although there was a degree of urgency but during the subsequent 4 years he developed normal control.

Postoperative shock

Postoperative shock occurred in a woman aged 22 years who presented with unilateral cavovarus foot and absent knee and ankle jerks; she had bad circulation in both lower limbs. A lipomatous tumour was found in the filum terminale near the conus and it was excised. The cause of the shock was possibly due to the release of tension in the spinal cord. She responded to treatment and made a very satisfactory recovery.

Wound infection

Early postoperative minor wound infection in the nature of a stitch abscess occurred in 5 of the cases but since the forty-seventh case there has been no instance of wound infection apart from 1 case which occurred 4 months after operation and was the result of late reaction to the sutures. Four cases responded to conservative treatment but in the case of delayed infection, excision of the wound edges and re-suture was necessary. When this work was started, silk was used as a routine for suturing, but after changing over to Mersilene no further cases of wound infection occurred apart from the single delayed case.

Cerebrospinal fluid fistula

Cerebrospinal fluid escaped from the wound postoperatively in 11 cases but was of a minor nature in 5 and rapidly subsided without treatment. In 3 cases the tiny dural defect through which the cerebrospinal fluid escaped was closed by re-suture.

In the other 3 cases repeated re-suturing did not control the leakage of cerebrospinal fluid and ventricular drainage had to be established; this needed to be maintained for at least 10 days before the leakage ceased and the wound healed, and the quantity of fluid discharged through the drain, together with the difficulty in controlling the flow from the fistula, suggested some abnormality of cerebrospinal fluid production. There was no other evidence, internal or external, to suggest that there was an associated Arnold–Chiari malformation. A cerebrospinal fluid fistula of this nature is dangerous because of the risk of meningitis but fortunately this complication did not occur in any of our cases.

If at any time in the postoperative period the dressing becomes moist with cerebrospinal fluid the wound must be inspected at once and the wound opened to repair the dural defect unless the leakage of cerebrospinal fluid is of a very minor nature. It must be emphasized that the leakage of cerebrospinal fluid must be stopped as soon as possible and if re-suture or fascial grafting is unsuccessful, ventricular drainage should be established and maintained for at least 10 days. In these cases, 6,000,000 I.U. of procaine penicillin are given by intramuscular injection before the child leaves the operating theatre; oral penicillin and sulphadimidine are given

6-hourly starting 12 hours after operation and continuing for at least 10 days.

This is a complication which cannot completely be avoided but we have reduced its incidence by suturing the dura mater with 0000 Mersilene on 20 mm half-circle eyeless round-bodied needles to make a watertight closure.

PART II

Analysis of 100 Cases
Submitted to Laminectomy

10—Reasons for Operation and Surgical Findings in General

Patients thought to be suffering from conditions associated with spina bifida occulta are referred by orthopaedic surgeons and other specialists to neurological surgeons. The symptoms presenting to these specialists are part of the syndrome but they are not always those which cause the neurological surgeon to decide to investigate further. Table 10.1 lists the categories of abnormality which were the principal reasons for establishing the need for myelography and laminectomy. Most cases suffered from more than one of these conditions: for example, Table 10.1 shows 14 cases of incontinence whereas there were 24 cases in the series which suffered from different degrees of bladder weakness. Here the principal conditions are classified and in later chapters information about individual abnormalities is elaborated.

TABLE 10.1

PRINCIPAL REASONS FOR OPERATION

Cavovarus, unilateral	26
Calcaneovalgus	4
Leg weakness	3
Monoplegia	11
Paraplegia	8
Incontinence	14
Trophic sepsis	12
Dermal sinus	3
Other abnormality	4
Clinically normal	15
	100

Unilateral cavovarus action and deformity was the clinical abnormality which originally drew our attention to the significance of spina bifida occulta. In the absence of reflex or sensory changes it is difficult to differentiate from the early stage of bilateral pes cavus or the effects of unperceived poliomyelitis and cases also occur for which no cause can be found. As with so many of the other presenting conditions, the existence of cutaneous abnormalities on the back indicated a possible cause; similarly, a suggestion of bladder weakness in the older child or adult was a guide.

Calcaneovalgus was unilateral in 3 cases and paretic in nature in all 4 cases. All had normal reflexes.

Leg weakness. The 3 cases are all difficult to classify. All had hypertrichosis, 1 with a lumbosacral lipoma; 2 had abnormal lower limb reflexes and 1 had a paralytic footdrop.

Monoplegia was manifested variously by limb weakness, spasticity or paralysis and sometimes accompanied by foot deformity. Bladder weakness was present in 1 case.

Paraplegia varied from minor degrees, through moderate spasticity to completely flail knees and ankles and was usually associated with incontinence.

Incontinence occurred alone in 5 cases, 3 of them adults; the remaining cases all had some foot abnormality as well, including 2 cases with relapsing bilateral congenital talipes enquinovarus.

Trophic sepsis was associated with foot deformities in all cases except one where the feet were normal but the boy had suffered from hot water bottle burns which were the first indication of any abnormality.

Dermal sinus. In all 3 cases there was a suggestion of discharge from the fistulous opening which in fact did not penetrate deeply except as a fibrosed solid cord. One child was incontinent but neither of the other cases had any other clinical abnormality.

Other abnormality. The 4 patients all had significant laminal defects and abnormalities demonstrated by myelography, 2 had relapsing club feet and abnormal reflexes, one had very poor circulation in the lower limbs and hypertrichosis, and the last, a woman aged 21 years, presented with sciatica, a contracture of one knee since early childhood and a wasted leg.

Clinically normal cases. Seven had lumbosacral lipomas. This is an abnormality which we believe should always be operated on (Chapter 15). All the patients had abnormal myelograms. Six had hypertrichosis which the parents were anxious to have removed. We considered that, before referring them to a plastic surgeon, it would be wise to exclude the possibility of laminal defects and myelographic abnormalities. Our argument is that if there is a spinal cord anomaly present, it may well produce a neurological deficit later on and laminectomy will be needed. The cosmetic surgery will necessitate two or three operations as the area of skin to be removed may be considerable and these operations may prejudice the patient against having a laminectomy later on if the occasion should arise. If the laminectomy is done first, the cosmetic surgery can follow if the psychological requirement persists. All 6 of these cases had significant laminal defects and abnormalities on myelography, 4 had diastematomyelia and 2 traction anomalies. The last 2 cases were each found to have a patch of thin pigmented naevoid skin after the hair had been shaved.

Both the other clinically normal cases required further investigation. One had a coccygeal cyst, and the other a naevoid patch on the back which was tender to touch; deep pressure or a blow produced a literally sickening pain, symptoms which caused the patient anxiety.

TABLE 10.2

FINDINGS AT OPERATION

Diastematomyelia—complete	41	p. 61
—partial	1	p. 75
Dermoid cysts	5	p. 77
Hydromyelia	2	p. 79
Myelodysplasia	2	p. 80
Pressure lesion	1	p. 80
Pressure and traction lesion	1	p. 80
Negative or ambiguous	1	p. 81
Traction lesions	71	p. 83
Filum terminale—tight	5	p. 84
—lipoma	1	p. 86
Dermal sinus	1	p. 87
Coccygeal cyst	2	p. 88
Meningocele manqué—true	11	p. 89
—possible	6	p. 93

A number of cases had more than one abnormality and they are accordingly classified under more than one heading.

Some of the abnormalities affecting the spinal cord in these cases have names which are familiar; the remainder are often too complicated to explain in a few words and are therefore grouped in Table 10.2 according to our conception of how they fit into the original three-group classification which we gave in our first publication on spinal dysraphism (James and Lassman, 1960). While basically correct, our classification is unpractical because it is difficult to know into which of these groups many of our cases should be placed; the same abnormality could exert traction at one time, pressure at another, or both at the same time. Of the named conditions, diastematomyelia with a bone septum is the best known and far too much stress is laid upon it. Only 17 per cent of our cases had a bone septum associated with diastematomyelia, which means that 83 per cent of cases of spina bifida occulta have some other abnormality affecting the spinal cord and nerve roots. All these conditions are discusssed in detail in the following chapters.

REFERENCE

James, C. C. M. and Lassman, L. P. (1960). 'Spinal Dysraphism.' *Archs. Dis. Childh.* **35**, 315.

11—Findings at Operation—I

DIASTEMATOMYELIA

Diastematomyelia is a bifid state of the spinal cord, an intrinsic anomaly and, being a form of myelodysplasia, requires no treatment. It results from a dorsiventral division of the neural tube in the embryo; its two halves are unequal in their cellular and neuronal content so that they represent neither two half spinal cords nor two spinal cords in parallel (which would constitute diplomyelia). The extent of the division may be minute, 1 or 2 mm longitudinally, or considerable, extending over very many segments. There may be several divisions in the one spinal cord. Usually, the two parts re-join caudally so that there is a single conus medullaris but there are cases where they do not do so. Williams and Nixon (1957) report 1 case and we also have 1 but not in this series. We have some doubt about this reunion of the spinal cord in our Case 15; the cauda equina on each side had its own dural sheath and its own sacral canal, there being sacral somatoschisis but we could not identify any filum terminale (*Figure 11.1*). Occasionally the division of the spinal cords is incomplete. Case 59 had separation of the dorsal spinal cord over a longitudinal length of 1·75 cm but the ventral parts were joined together in what appeared to be the normal manner; there was a single dural tube (p. 75).

There are two principal reasons for the clinical importance of diastematomyelia; first, there may be a septum passing dorsiventrally between the two spinal cords and secondly there may be what we can only call bands arising from one or both spinal cords which attach to the internal surface of the dura mater or pass through to attach externally to a neural arch or to the subcutaneous tissues. Both septum and bands may occur together or in cases with multiple divisions of the spinal cord there may be bands and more than one septum at different levels together or separately.

61

Importance of a septum

The septum may be of bone, cartilage, fibrous tissue or a mixture of these; it passes dorsiventrally between the dorsal surface of one or more vertebral bodies and the neural arches so making locally two vertebral canals. It is rare for a septum not to be complete in this way although the point of junction either dorsally or ventrally may be very fine and tenuous. At the site of a septum, we have always found a complete ossified neural arch although the spinous process may not be well formed; laminal defects of spina bifida are in neighbouring neural arches. With one exception, all the cases of diastematomyelia with septum that we have operated on have also had two

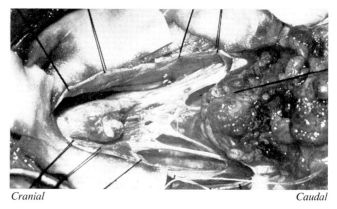

Cranial   Caudal

Figure 11.1: Case 15. Dura mater opened to show two terminal sacs each containing half of the cauda equina; between is a saddle of bone and fibrous fatty tissue. The stalk of the subcutaneous lipoma has been removed from the conus medullaris seen in the centre (Lv3 level)

dural sheaths (or tubes) visible on inspection after removal of the laminae. In all cases there have been two layers of the dura mater as well as the septum between the two spinal cords. The exceptional case had a septum attaching to a vertebral body at one extremity and at the other to the internal surface of the dura mater dorsally so that there was no extradural evidence of the two dural tubes within (James and Lassman, 1967). This exceptional case is not in this series (*Figure 11.2*); there were two septa as well as bands.

The importance of the septum is that it may be placed at or near the caudal point of junction (bifurcation) of the two spinal cords so that during the so-called ascent of the spinal cord owing to relatively greater growth in length of the vertebral column, considerable pressure is borne by the bifurcation with consequent interference with nerve conduction or blood supply. There may also be pressure necrosis of cells. The septum may also cause lateral pressure on one of the spinal cords with similar results (*Figure 11.3*). Furthermore, in early childhood there may be sufficient space in the two local vertebral canals to accommodate the spinal cords but with growth and maturation, not only will the spinal cords themselves increase in bulk but the walls of the vertebral canal may thicken and narrow the

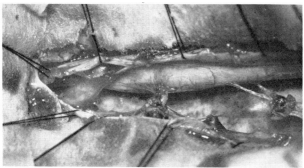

Cranial   Figure 11.2   *Caudal*

Figure 11.2: Case not in this series. Dura mater opened. Right spinal cord clearly seen with intrathecal septum (Tv10) crossing it at the left end of the exposure, the left spinal cord is hidden under the near edge of the dura. In the centre is a commissural band (Tv12) between the two spinal cords. To the right is the base of the septum at Lv2

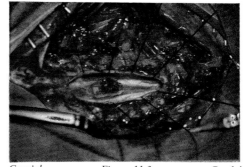

Figure 11.3: Case 9. Dura mater open. Diastemato- myelia with a bone septum (Tv9). Note cut edges of the dura mater around the bony septum. The septum causing pressure on the right half of the spinal cord

Cranial   Figure 11.3   *Caudal*

canals. In all this the dural part of the septum is inert but when the septum is removed surgically, the dura mater must be removed as well otherwise it remains as a cause of pressure, a preventive of movement and possibly of expansion of the spinal cord later (*Figure 11.4*).

There is no satisfactory explanation for the pressure caused by a septum on the caudal junction of the two spinal cords because symptoms occur late rather than at birth when the conus medullaris has normally attained its final vertebral level. Barson (1970) suggests that the normal ascent of the spinal cord is unusually retarded in cases of diastematomyelia or that the ascent is slowed but not prevented and therefore continues into childhood beyond the normal time of cessation; because of the ability of immature neuronal tissue

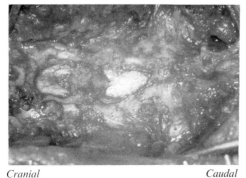

Figure 11.4: Case 14

(a) *Extradural appearances. Bone septum is in the centre with the dura mater cranial and caudal to it. The latter is bulging and shiny in comparison with the healthy dura cranial to the septum*

Cranial   *Caudal*

(b) *Dura mater opened. The bone septum and surrounding dura mater have been removed. The septum was closely adherent to the caudal junction of the two spinal cords and the caudal part appears engorged with blood in comparison with the cranial portion*

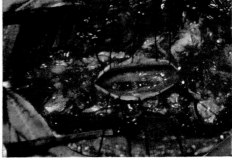

Cranial   *Caudal*

to develop alternative pathways, neurological damage is not evident clinically until this capacity is slowly lost during early childhood. Similarly, Barson's second explanation might be thought to apply in cases where the spinal cord is pressed upon by a narrowing bone tube. It would otherwise be thought that maturing spinal cord would not increase in volume locally in an area where the surrounding bone was thickening and narrowing the channel; failure to myelinate normally in such a situation might account for unsatisfactory neuronal conduction.

The chance finding of a bone septum during examination for some other condition than spina bifida is not a direct reason for its immediate surgical removal. The patient will need to be watched carefully for evidence of neurological deficit. Similarly, it has been our practice in cases needing operation and which have more than one area of diastematomyelia to explore the more caudal area, watching subsequent progress in case a further exploration at a higher level should become necessary. Case 86 was such a patient (p. 129). It may be wiser to remove a bone septum discovered adventitiously because there is no means of determining its relation to a point of union of the two spinal cords except by direct exploration; a myelogram can only demonstrate the existence of the septum, it cannot reliably indicate the extent of the diastematomyelia or the situation of the bifurcations. The septum and the two dural sheaths usually occupy only a small part of the hiatus between the two spinal cords. However, it is possible for diastematomyelia with a septum to exist throughout life without giving rise to trouble of any kind. Our morbid anatomy research provided us with autopsy Case 137 (p. 22), a woman of 64 who died of cerebral thrombosis following cardiac infarction and who had no neurological deficit or lower limb abnormality on admission to hospital. She had diastematomyelia with a bone septum at Lv4 level and her conus medullaris was immediately caudal to this. The septum and dural tubes were very small and fitted tightly into the hiatus between the two spinal cords.

In Chapter 3, when discussing this case, we postulated that the possibility of a septum not causing spinal cord injury might be related to its site and its distance from the conus medullaris because these factors might affect the ability of the spinal cord to grow sufficiently to prevent any traction effect. In this series of cases operated upon, there were 6 in which the septum was clearly pressing on the caudal bifurcation of the spinal cord, details are as follows.

Case No.	Age (years)	Septum level	Length of hiatus (cm)	Conus level	Result after laminectomy
14	6	Tv12	2·5	Lv2	Improved (p. 133)
36	3	Lv2	2·0	Lv4	Still normal
52	10¾	Lv3	3·5	Lv5	Unchanged
57	5	Lv2	2·5	Lv3	Unchanged
58	1¼	Lv4	1·5	Sv1	Possibly improved (p. 131)
97	21	Lv2	2·0	Lv4	Unchanged

Case 36 (*Figure 11.5*) was clinically normal but had hypertrichosis; the remainder all had unilateral neurological deficit.

This information is inconclusive. It would appear that in every case the septum was at a greater distance from the conus medullaris than was the situation in autopsy Case 137, particularly when consideration is given to the vertebral body size at the different ages; Case 57 is the only one in doubt in this respect. It could be thought that the more caudal the septum was situated, the more likely the greater length of the spinal cord cranially would be able to accommodate to the slowly increasing tension but these 6 cases with the pressure effect do not provide sufficient evidence in this respect. It is quite possible that the reason for the absence of pressure in our postmortem case was that the spinal cord had been absolutely fixed without any possibility of movement from about 4 weeks after conception and for 64 years of life. The tension of growth was therefore continuous and the neural tissue had been able to develop normally. In our clinical cases the spinal cord had not been under steady tension and when the traction force became effective its onset was too rapid and too forcible for the tissues to be able to respond by growth. In all our other clinical cases, there was none with a close fit by the spinal cord around the septum. In the remaining 14 cases the site of the septum and of the conus medullaris was as follows.

Site of septum		Site of conus medullaris
Tv9	1 case	Not identified
Tv11	1 case	Lv3/4, by myelography
Tv12	1 case	Lv3, by myelography
Lv2	3 cases	Lv4 in 2 cases, Lv5 in 1 case
Lv3	4 cases	Lv4 in 3 cases, Lv5 in 1 case
	2 cases	Lv4/5 and Sv1, both by myelography
Lv4	1 case	Sv1
Lv5	1 case	Sv1

In some cases the conus medullaris was not seen at operation; their site is shown as determined by myelography.

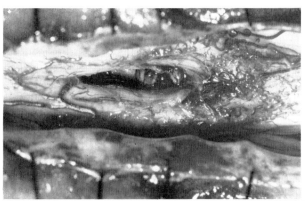

Cranial *Caudal*

Figure 11.5: Case 36. Dura mater open. The bone septum (Lv3) and the median dura have been removed. Diastematomyelia is in the centre; the bone septum had occupied the caudal half and had been pressing on the spinal cord which is swollen and engorged (to the right of the photograph) as compared with the normal spinal cord (to the left)

One case (9) aged 13 years had lateral pressure from the septum on one spinal cord (*Figure 11.3*), and one (6) aged 13 years had dorsal pressure on both spinal cords from the fatty fibrous tissue which replaced the laminae immediately caudal to the septum. Both of these cases have improved following operation.

In the 41 cases of diastematomyelia in our series of 100 cases, a septum was present in 20 of which 16 were bone, 3 were fibrous and 1 was mixed, for example, 3 areas of diastematomyelia, 1 with a bone septum, 1 with a fibrous septum and 1 with no septum, the spinal cord was apparently fully reconstituted between each segment of diastematomyelia and not simply joined by the commissural bands discussed in the next section (Table 11.1).

TABLE 11.1

DIASTEMATOMYELIA—41 CASES

Septum—bone	16	
—fibrous	3	19
No septum		21
Mixed*		1

* 3 areas of diastematomyelia: bone septum, fibrous septum, no septum.

Importance of bands

This is an objectionable term but we can find no other simple terminology. These bands up to 0·5 cm diameter are commonly aberrant dorsal nerve roots. This has been shown by microscopy of specimens removed at operation; other specimens of approximately the same or slightly less diameter, have consisted of dense fibrous tissue and we postulate that some of the latter are nerve roots formed in the embryo which failed to find a functional path and so atrophied. Some of the bands are minute in cross-section but they have a considerable tensile strength and because they run singly and not in multiples they cannot be simple adhesions. All these bands are found outside the dura mater as well as inside, usually in continuity. Occasionally we have found them only extradurally, occasionally only intradurally and presumably their other end has been concealed or destroyed during the surgical approach. When there are several bands in any one case they seem to occur segmentally, one band arising from one interlaminar area, one band from the next and so on; they are often accompanied by blood vessels. Where the bands are fibrous, the possibility of meningocele manqué arises (Chapter 14).

In general, in diastematomyelia these bands run between the neural arch joints, that is, interlaminar or interspinous process or from the fatty fibrous tissue which substitutes for bone in defective neural arches, and continue through the dura mater at a more cranial level to pass intrathecally to attach to the spinal cord or the cauda equina, normally more cranial to the point of penetration of the dura mater. However, occasionally, the band may turn caudally

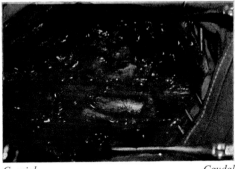

(a) *Extradural band (elevated by probe) emerging from beneath the neural arch of Lv1 to attach to the dura mater at the level of Tv11*

Cranial   Caudal

(b) *Dura mater opened. The traction band has been divided extradurally, its dural end lying on the swab lining near side of wound. Intradural extension of the band is seen passing caudally to attach to the spinal cord in the midline just below the point of union of the bifid spinal cord (Tv12). There is no septum. Forceps hold cut edge of an arachnoid veil which passed across the hiatus of the diastematomyelia to be attached to the intrathecal part of the band which was an ectopic dorsal nerve root*

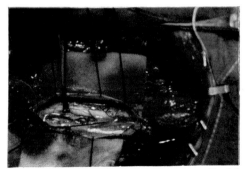

Cranial   Caudal

Figure 11.6: Case 12

after passing through the dura mater (*Figures 11.6, 11.7*). Within the theca they commonly attach to one or other bifurcation of the spinal cord, one band to each, and others may join bands which pass between the two spinal cords: these we term commissural bands since this would seem to be their function and possibly is the means whereby spinal cord tracts cross from one spinal cord to the other (*Figure 11.8*). Occasionally, a band may be attached to a loop of recurrent nerve roots or nerves which arise from the spinal cord and re-enter the spinal cord again. These bands have a different origin from those mentioned previously; they are almost certainly remnants of a meningocele which actually failed to form or, having formed, atrophied (Chapter 14). Such bands are always seen to be fibrous on microscopy and rarely associated with a blood vessel. Bands most commonly occur in cases of diastematomyelia without a septum, usually one segment away, and we have found them in cases without diastematomyelia. Their importance lies in their tethering or traction

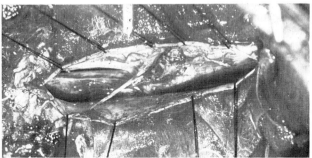

Cranial   Caudal

Figure 11.7: Case 24. Dura mater opened. An extradural band extended vertically from Lv2 neural arch to attach to the dura and continued intrathecally in a caudal direction. Intrathecal part only is shown left of centre, passing to the right of the exposure (Lv3 and 4 level). No septum

effect upon the intrathecal structures. Their obliquity, starting at one neural arch and passing cranially 2 or 3 segments before penetrating the dura, indicates that they have a capacity for growth but some are obviously pulling the spinal cord dorsally against the dura mater in a caudal direction; when the band is cut there is immediate retraction of the neural tissue which falls to lie in a more normal relationship to other structures. In one case the two spinal cords of diastemato-myelia without septum were held widely apart by a band and after release the hiatus between the two spinal cords was no longer visible. Table 11.2 shows that severing these bands can produce definite results.

TABLE 11.2

SINGLE DURAL TUBE—21 CASES: RESULT OF OPERATION ON 15 CASES WITH BANDS

Before operation	No. of cases	After operation (follow-up 2–7 years)
Reflexes normal	1	Reflexes normal, no further deterioration in gait or foot shape
Reflexes abnormal	4	One or more reflexes changed to normal
	7	Reflexes unchanged, gait improved
	3*	Reflexes unchanged, no further deterioration in gait or foot shape

* Case 60 subsequently developed rheumatoid arthritis.
Six cases of diastematomyelia with a single dural tube did not have bands.

Various theories have been advanced for the cause of diastematomyelia; one suggested that the condition was associated with in-
turning of the laminae to form a septum. This theory can be
discounted on several grounds but it is true that the laminae can be
inverted, that is, rotated on their transverse axis so that one margin
(usually the cranial edge) presses down into the vertebral canal
against the dura and underlying structures. When a lamina is
inverted in this way and the intrathecal nervous tissue is tightly held
up against it by a band, there must be both pressure and traction on
the nervous tissue. We have had at least one case of this type (30)
with outstanding clinical improvement following operation.

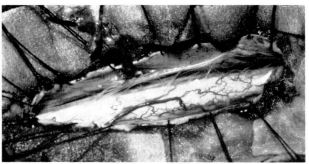

Cranial   Caudal

*Figure 11.8: Case 51. Dura mater open. Diastematomyelia seen
throughout the exposure: neither bifurcation is shown. In the centre is
a nerve passing from the left to the right where it penetrates the dura
(Lv2). It receives contributions from both spinal cords and at its origin
it lies over and conceals commissural bands which are connected
through the dura to the neural arch of Lv1; this connection can be
seen left of centre lying upon the surrounding swabs. There was a third
similar band from the neural arch of Tv12 which is not shown. The
two spinal cords were of equal size although the photograph suggests
that the left one was very large*

Table 11.3 shows the findings at operation in the 21 cases where the
diastematomyelia was contained within a single dural tube and there
was no septum.

The 2 cases classed in Table 11.3 as having no extrinsic abnormality both had diastematomyelia in a single dural tube and no
septum. Case 17 (*Figure 11.9*) was notable in having dorsal nerve
roots originating on the left spinal cord near the median dorsal
margin which passed across the right spinal cord to leave the vertebral canal with right-sided ventral nerve roots. Case 98 was similar
but much more complicated: the right spinal cord was three times
the bulk of the left spinal cord, the caudal bifurcation formed the

TABLE 11.3

Band connecting to spinal cord		
from neural arch	11	
from dura mater	3	
	—	14
Band connected to filum terminale		1
No bands		
Filum terminale adherent to one side and rotating the spinal cord	1	
Conus medullaris adherent to dura mater and compressed by inverted laminae	1	
Multiple intradural adhesions of spinal cord	1	
Lipomatous plug between spinal cords connecting to subcutaneous tissues	1	
	—	4
No extrinsic abnormality affecting spinal cord		2

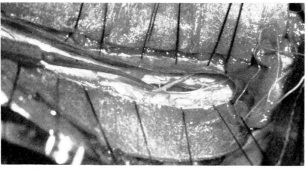

Cranial Caudal

Figure 11.9: Case 17. Dura mater open. Diastematomyelia with caudal bifurcation at right. There is a dorsal nerve root originating from the left spinal cord passing across the dorsum of the right spinal cord to join the latter's ventral root. A similar smaller root is seen more caudally crossing the bifurcation to pass out of the right side of the theca

conus medullaris at the termination of the dural sac under the neural arch Sv2/3, and there was no identifiable filum terminale; it could not have existed within the dura as there was no space for it. Several nerve roots originating from the dorsum of the right spinal cord passed over the left one and joined the left side ventral nerve roots; their course was that seen in the foetus, at right angles to the spinal cord and without obliquity. The diastematomyelia occupied the full length of the exposure and the cranial bifurcation could not be seen.

In this section we have made only passing reference to the bands of a different type which are referred to in Chapter 15 on cases of lumbosacral lipoma, of pigmented naevi, of dermal dimples and sinuses and (in Chapter 14) meningocele manqué.

CLINICAL SYNDROMES

Table 11.4 shows the clinical syndromes associated with diastematomyelia. There is no relation between these different groups and the type of abnormality found at operation but this table does not give

TABLE 11.4

DIASTEMATOMYELIA: CLINICAL SYNDROME IN 41 CASES

Normal apart from cutaneous manifestation	4
Short leg with neurological deficit	4
Short leg without neurological deficit	1
Short foot without neurological deficit	2
Short foot and leg without neurological deficit	3
Short foot and leg with neurological deficit	19
Abnormal feet with neurological deficit	6
Normal feet with neurological deficit	1
Incontinence, normal lower limbs	1

There is no relationship with the clinical findings of the presence or absence of a septum.

TABLE 11.5

DIASTEMATOMYELIA: CUTANEOUS ABNORMALITIES IN 41 CASES

Hypertrichosis		
with naevus	6	
with lipoma	3	
with lipoma and naevus	1	
alone	10	
	—	20
Lipoma		
with naevus	3	
alone	1	
	—	4
Naevus alone		1
Dermal dimple		4
		29
No cutaneous abnormality		12

The incidence of hypertrichosis is 48 per cent of cases of diastematomyelia as compared with 39 per cent of all cases in this series.

a full indication of the incidence of external cutaneous manifestations which were found in 29 cases. These are shown in Table 11.5 and the frequency of hypertrichosis needs to be commented on particularly since it has been said to be indicative of diastematomyelia. The incidence appears to be high, 20 out of 41 cases (48 per cent) of diastematomyelia as compared with 39 per cent for the whole series of 100 cases reported here. As mentioned in Chapter 15 on cutaneous abnormalities, there are 3 types of hypertrichosis but analysis does not show any one of them as being particularly associated with diastematomyelia or any other type of spinal cord anomaly.

DISCUSSION

Diastematomyelia was a word originally coined by Hertwig to describe a condition where the spinal cord developed in two parts and with a gap between them. In clinical discussion and on reading the literature one gains the impression that to many clinicians diastematomyelia is a name for a bone septum dividing the vertebral canal dorsiventrally. The word has even been used in relation to bone septa in the sacral region; diastematomyelia as originally coined is impossible in the cauda equina. The fact that two spinal cords can exist without any septum is either ignored or has been overshadowed by the much more easily diagnosed cases which have a septum. This separation into two identities is made more emphatic because some writers insist that in the absence of a septum the condition is one of diplomyelia, implying that there is duplication of the spinal cord. This latter term was brought into prominence by Herren and Edwards (1940) who used it because they said it implied a more or less perfect duplication of the spinal cord and their illustrative case certainly goes some way to justify their opinion. However, in their review of the literature they provided information about a further 42 cases of which at least 7 had a septum. Since diplomyelia in the sense in which it is used by Herren and Edwards can only be diagnosed by transection of the spinal cord it should be avoided in a clinical environment. Lichtenstein (1940) in referring to a case preferred diastematomyelia to diplomyelia because the condition was not a true duplication but a diastasis of one spinal cord into two parts. Throughout our work therefore we have avoided the term diplomyelia and used diastematomyelia although it is admittedly cumbersome to have to associate the word with the presence or absence of a septum. From an examination of our records, we can find nothing to distinguish one type of diastematomyelia from the other (that is, with or without a septum) in respect to clinical syndromes or prognosis but they probably result from the same type of embryological defect with slight differences of time of onset, duration and severity of the causal agent.

The Herren and Edwards (1940) case demonstrated very clearly the 90° rotation of the spinal cords, the variation in the central canal and the distribution of the white and grey matter. In the other cases they discussed, mention is made of several in which each spinal cord was associated with 4 primary nerve roots, a pair of ventral and dorsal roots lying laterally and a pair situated medially. In most of these cases, however, the lateral roots were well formed, while the medial, when present, were rudimentary and were associated with under-developed grey columns. In our cases we have not found pairs of medial roots, but only single fairly well formed nerves which from their point of origin it was thought were dorsal roots; they could of course have been ventral roots as we had not considered the rotation of the spinal cord which occurs with diastematomyelia. When present in our cases, these medial roots have passed across the other spinal cord to join the outgoing nerve roots on the other side except in one case where a single medial root passed ventrally to the other spinal cord. Saunders (1943) illustrates a case in which sets of roots arose from both medial and lateral aspects of one spinal cord and joined to produce a medial and a lateral set of nerves. Dorsal and ventral nerve roots with an origin from the median aspect of a spinal cord do not seem to be common in reported cases and we have neither seen a case of our own nor found one mentioned in the literature where median roots occurred on both spinal cords: the roots always seem to emerge from only one of them.

Matson and colleagues (1950) in their account of diastemato-myelia, its diagnosis and treatment, brought the subject to general attention and stated their preference for the word diastematomyelia as opposed to diplomyelia. Their masterly coverage of the subject has impressed very widely and because they made no mention of diastematomyelia without a septum, readers seem to have assumed that diastematomyelia is a septum. We note with interest that two of their cases had 'small dermoid inclusion cysts in the spinal canal at a level adjacent to the diastematomyelia'. One of our cases had such a cyst in a laminal defect as also did one of our cases of lumbo-sacral lipoma.

In all our cases of diastematomyelia with septum we have found a more or less complete neural arch associated; the laminae are not perfectly formed and the major laminal defects have been in neigh-bouring neural arches. Perret (1960) describes 2 cases where only one of a pair of laminae was present and this was connected to the

74

septum. In 1 of these cases a dorsal nerve root passed dorsally through the bone septum to cross over the other spinal cord and join the outgoing ventral nerve root on that side; this median nerve root was preserved during removal of the septum. Perret recommends dividing the filum terminale in order to make sure that there is no longer any traction effect. This has not been our practice: commonly, the conus medullaris is not exposed at operation and in many cases the filum terminale is a very broad structure because it almost always incorporates nerve roots of the cauda equina. Where the filum terminale has been visibly tight, we have dissected off these nerve roots before cutting the filum within the field of operation taking the risk of destroying their blood supply. But we prefer to cut it near to its attachment to the terminal dural sac. In spite of our caution, material taken at the time shows on microscopy that we have always cut small nerves in removing the fragment.

We have discussed diastematomyelia as being a dorsiventral division of the spinal cord and this is how other authors have regarded the condition, yet it is interesting to note that Warkany (1960) in his experimental work on the production of malformations of the central nervous system has repeatedly produced division of the spinal cord but always transversely (a dorsal and a ventral cord) and never dorsiventrally. This transverse division has, however, been found by chance at human autopsy and it is possible that such a condition was developing in the embryo described by Gruenwald (1941).

PARTIAL DIASTEMATOMYELIA

Case 59, a boy aged $2\frac{1}{2}$ years, is referred to on p. 61. He was operated on because of hypertrichosis and an indefinably abnormal use of one foot with some loss of power in this limb; there did not appear to be any sensory loss. At operation, there were strong adhesions between the dura mater and the last 3 cm of the spinal cord on each side and also in the midline dorsally. The midline adhesions resembled a septum dividing the dural tube into two halves at Lv3/4 level; when cut away from their spinal cord attachment, the adhesions were seen to be attached on each side to the two spinal cords of diastematomyelia but deeper examination showed that the two spinal cords were joined ventrally. All the adhesions were divided so that the spinal cord was freed from fixation. Seven years after operation, the boy was clinically normal.

REFERENCES

Barson, A. J. (1970). 'The Vertebral Level of Termination of the Spinal Cord during Normal and Abnormal Development.' *J. Anat.* **106**, 489

Gruenwald, P. (1941). 'Tissue Anomalies of Probable Neural Crest Origin in Twenty Millimeter Human Embryo with Myeloschisis.' *Archs. Path.* **31**, 489

Herren, R. Y. and Edwards, J. E. (1940). 'Diplomyelia (Duplication of the Spinal Cord).' *Archs. Path.* **30**, 1203

James, C. C. M. and Lassman, L. P. (1964). 'Diastematomyelia. A Critical Survey of 24 Cases Submitted to Laminectomy.' *Archs. Dis. Childh.* **39**, 125

— — (1967). 'Diastematomyelia in Spina Bifida Occulta. A Report of an Unusual Finding at Operation.' *Folia psychiat. neurol. neurochir. neerl.* **70**, 453

— — (1970). 'Diastematomyelia and Tight Filum Terminale.' *J. Neurol. Sci.* **10**, 193

Matson, D. D., Woods, R. P., Campbell, J. B. and Ingraham, F. D. (1950). 'Diastematomyelia (Congenital Clefts of the Spinal Cord). Diagnosis and Surgical Treatment.' *Pediatrics, Springfield* **6**, 98

Perret, G. (1960). 'Symptoms and Diagnosis of Diastematomyelia.' *Neurology, Minneap.* **10**, 51

Saunders, R. L. de C. H. (1943). 'Combined Anterior and Posterior Spina Bifida in a Living Neonatal Human Female.' *Anat. Rec.* **87**, 255

Warkany, J. (1960). 'Experimental Production of Congenital Malformations of the Central Nervous System.' *Proceedings 1st Int. Conf. on Mental Retardation*, pp. 44–64. Ed. by P. W. Bowman and H. V. Mautner. New York; Grune and Stratton

Williams, D. I. and Nixon, H. H. (1957). 'Agenesis of the Sacrum.' *Surgery Gynec. Obstet.* **105**, 84

12—Findings at Operation—II

DERMOID CYSTS

In 3 cases the cyst was intramedullary and in 2 it was situated amongst the cauda equina.

Cyst intramedullary

In Case 95, a woman aged 44 years, although the cyst was within the spinal cord and conus medullaris overlying the region of Lv1 and 2 vertebral bodies, it was possible to excise it apparently completely and to break down the local adhesions. She had a history of incontinence of 5 years' duration and increasing weakness of one lower limb; the former is unchanged so that a ureteric diversion has been performed but she had regained almost normal power in her leg 2 years later.

In Cases 70 and 99 it was impossible to remove the cyst so that in the former it was emptied by aspiration and in the latter by direct incision. In Case 70, it was situated in the spinal cord extending over Tv12–Lv2 levels, the conus being at Lv3. In Case 99, the cyst was very extensive, from Tv8–Lv4 and involved the conus medullaris which was expanded to extend to a lower level than the situation of the nerve root origins of the cauda equina suggested that it had been originally. Case 70 was a girl aged $2\frac{1}{4}$ years who presented with incontinence, a condition which has improved to allow normal control during the subsequent 6 years; but she is still occasionally troubled by urinary infection. Case 99, a boy aged $3\frac{1}{2}$ years presented with severe and progressive weakness of a leg which is now much stronger and with total incontinence which continues unchanged 5 years later.

Cyst in cauda equina

Of the 2 cases in which the cyst was situated in the cauda equina, Case 31 had had a dermal fistula excised superficially at the age of

$3\frac{1}{2}$ years because of recurrent meningitis which had not subsequently recurred but he presented to us with moderate spasticity of both lower limbs and with retention and overflow of urine. At operation, the fibrosis associated with the dermoid cyst was extensive and involved all the nerve roots so that it could only be opened by direct incision and emptied. As a result, he lost his spasticity but continues, 8 years later, with his lack of urinary control. In Case 67, however, it was possible to remove the cyst complete including the terminal portion attached to the conus medullaris; the filum terminale had to be cut to permit this but it was not clear whether the cyst was within the filum or only attached to it. Aged 9 years at the time of laminectomy, his clinical state is unaltered 5 years later; he continues to be totally incontinent and to have paretic valgoid feet with some foot-drop.

In all these cases, examination of the material removed confirmed the diagnosis. Where solid material was obtained, the cysts were lined by stratified squamous epithelium and had hair follicles; where only fluid was obtained it contained squames. All the cysts were sterile.

Survey radiographic examination showed multiple laminal defects in Cases 31, 67 and 70. In Case 95 only Sv1 laminae were abnormal and in Case 99 only Lv5.

DISCUSSION

According to Manno, Uihlein and Kernohan (1962), dermoids differ from epidermoids in that they contain hair, sebaceous glands and other appendages of skin whereas epidermoids have no hair or sebaceous glands. By that standard only 2 of our cases had a dermoid cyst and the other 3 had epidermoids. Manno and colleagues reviewed 90 reported cases with epidermoids but excluded 37 cases as being non-congenital: they resulted from skin puncture implantation. None of our 5 cases had had lumbar punctures performed but 1 had had a dermal sinus excised at a previous operation. The third group of Manno's cases, 6 in number, had a communicating dermal sinus but the cysts were extramedullary. In the whole series of 53 cases accepted as having epidermoids of congenital origin, 19 were intra-medullary and 34 were situated in the thoracic spinal region.

Willis (1958) states that the subdivision of sequestrated skin-lined cysts into dermoids and epidermoids is pointless because the differential depends on minutiae and the case reported by Kirsch and Hodges (1966) confirms this contention. Their case of epidermoid was macroscopically a dermoid because it contained hair and

78

desquamated skin whereas microscopy revealed no hair follicles and only desquamated skin and atrophied epithelium consistent with an epidermoid.

The cholesterol content of intrathecal epidermoids is said to be irritating and Decker and Gross (1967) report a case of a ruptured cyst lying amongst the cauda equina which presented with meningitic symptoms. The child had had headache and abdominal pain following a fall from a bicycle and a few days later developed meningitic symptoms and signs. The authors considered that the cyst material had caused a chemical meningitis but microscopy did not demonstrate the presence of cholesterol. Manno, Uihlein and Kernohan (1962) considered this subject with care and analysis showed that in 4 epidermoid cysts the cholesterol content was negligible but that the fat content was considerable. In none of our 5 cases was cholesterol seen on microscopy.

Two more of our cases had dermoids in defective laminae. In Case 39 the cyst was found while following the deep connection of a lumbosacral lipoma to the point where it plugged an intradural myelocele; the dermoid was at dural level caudal to the point where the lipoma connection entered the dura mater. In Case 65, the cyst was associated with defective laminae at Lv5 level in a case with diastematomyelia without septum situated at Lv2/3 level.

HYDROMYELIA

These 2 cases have been previously reported (Lassman, James and Foster, 1968). In Case 35, the hydromyelia was noted in the spinal cord (Tv12/Lv1 level) at the cranial bifurcation of diastematomyelia with an osseo-fibrous septum over Lv2/3 disc; the cystic swelling was aspirated to give about 1·25 ml of clear fluid which, however, was not investigated for protein content. There was a further diastematomyelia, starting 1·5 cm caudally, without a septum.

In Case 91, the diagnosis was made on clinical grounds, radiography showed laminal defects in the region of Tv1–8 and cisternal myelography demonstrated an incomplete obstruction to the downward flow of Myodil at Cv6 level. At laminectomy, the spinal cord was seen to be expanded and very thin walled from Cv6 to Tv8; the cystic swelling was incised in its midline and the clear fluid content sucked away. He was a boy aged 1½ years with a history of increasing spinal muscle weakness and partial left foot-drop; the left knee jerk was diminished and the ankle jerk was absent. Following a fall on his buttocks he became very weak in both lower limbs so that he was hardly able to stand. Four years after laminectomy his left knee and ankle jerks are absent but his strength has returned and he appears a normal boy apart from a mild high cervicothoracic kyphosis.

Nassar, Correll and Housepian (1968) report 3 cases of intra-medullary cystic lesions of the conus medullaris 2 of which were probably developmental errors in the formation of the ventriculus terminalis of the conus medullaris, the third case could also have been of similar origin but there was a connection with the central canal of the spinal cord as well as myelographic evidence of expansion of the cervicothoracic spinal cord which suggests that the cyst in this case was a form of hydromyelia. We have subsequently encountered a case (Lassman, James and Foster, 1968) where there was a cystic enlargement of the conus medullaris which pulsated rhythmically; it contained clear fluid resembling cerebrospinal fluid.

MYELODYSPLASIA

Cases 62 and 22 were both found at laminectomy to have a bulbous non-cystic enlargement of the terminal spinal cord and conus medullaris which was covered by large and tortuous blood vessels. In each case, the conus medullaris was situated at an abnormally low level, Lv5 in one, Lv3 in the other. In the latter, there was also an extradural fibrous band from the neural arch of Lv5 attaching to the dura mater at Lv4 level but no deeper connection could be found.

The younger, a boy aged 18 months, had a mild paraparesis which has slowly improved as also has his bladder control during the 7 years after laminectomy. The older, a girl aged nearly 7 years continues unchanged with absent left lower limb reflexes but with greater limb strength 8 years after laminectomy. Both children had multiple laminal defects in the lower lumbar region and sacrum; neither had skin evidence of underlying abnormality.

PRESSURE LESIONS AND PRESSURE WITH TRACTION

There was one case of each, both have been previously reported in detail (James and Lassman, 1960, Cases 2 and 14). The pressure abnormality in each case was a ligamentous transverse band intrinsic with the dura mater; the traction element of the second case was a band from the fatty fibrous tissue occupying the area of the unformed laminae of Lv5 and Sv1 which divided into fine strands to join the caudal edge of the transverse band which was pulled caudally and to the right side. In this latter case (8), the underlying spinal cord was of normal appearance but had been pressed upon cranial to the conus medullaris; in the former case (2) the transverse band had grooved the spinal cord which showed a reactionary enlargment both cranial and caudal to the transverse pressure area.

Both patients have made great improvement in the years since laminectomy. Case 8 with the pressure and traction lesion has normally shaped feet, the previously affected one being 1 cm shorter. His reflexes are unchanged, the left plantar response continuing to be extensor. Three and a half years after laminectomy, an operation was done to lengthen the left achilles tendon but otherwise he has required no orthopaedic care. Sensation and sphincter control are normal (10 years follow up).

Case 2 who had become almost flail in his lower limbs by the time of laminectomy at the age of 4 years has recovered good muscle function, wears a caliper on his right lower limb and enjoys playing football in leisure time. He has recovered bowel and bladder sensation but has little control. There continues to be absence of sensation in his tibiae and feet; he has fractured one tibia twice without suffering any pain (13 years follow-up).

NEGATIVE OPERATION FINDING

Case 11, a girl aged $12\frac{1}{2}$ years, presented with a painful enlarged fifth toe and early cavovarus deformity of the left foot. The ankle jerk was absent and the plantar response extensor; there was also anaesthesia to cotton wool over the outer 3 toes and the outer border of the foot. The myelogram appearances were ambiguous and this being an early case in our series, the conus medullaris was not identified. At laminectomy Lv4–Sv1, the conus medullaris was cranial to the area exposed and the cauda equina appeared normal; the dura mater was thickened at the lumbosacral level by a band of oblique ligamentous fibres very much thicker at their caudal edge and narrowing the intrathecal space. Six and a half years later, the cavovarus deformity and area of anaesthesia were unchanged and the plantar response was flexor. The patient has not been available for review since then.

REFERENCES

Decker, R. E. and Gross, S. W. (1967). 'Intraspinal Dermoid Tumor Presenting as Chemical Meningitis. Report of a Case Without Dermal Sinus.' *J. Neurosurg.* **27**, 60

James, C. C. M. and Lassman, L. P. (1960). 'Spinal Dysraphism.' *Archs. Dis. Childh.* **35**, 315

Kirsch, W. M. and Hodges, F. J. (1966). 'An Intramedullary Epidermal Inclusion Cyst of the Thoracic Cord Associated with a Previously Repaired Meningocoele.' *J. Neurosurg.* **24**, 1018

Lassman, L. P., James, C. C. M. and Foster, J. B. (1968). 'Hydromyelia.' *J. Neurol. Sci.* **7**, 149

Manno, N. J., Uihlein, A. and Kernohan, J. W. (1962). 'Intraspinal Epidermoids.' *J. Neurosurg.* **19**, 754

Nassar, S. I., Correll, J. W. and Housepian, E. M. (1968). 'Intramedullary Cystic Lesions of the Conus Medullaris.' *J. Neurol. Neurosurg. Psychiat.* **31**, 106

Willis, R. A. (1958). *The Borderland of Embryology and Pathology*, p. 307. London; Butterworths

13—Findings at Operation—III

TRACTION LESIONS

Cases with traction lesions are those having abnormalities which we believe tether the intrathecal nervous tissue so that ascent within the vertebral canal is prevented during growth or the maturation of fibrous tissue causes tension when the fibrous tissue has contracted into its final state. These abnormalities are bands or adhesions within

TABLE 13.1

TRACTION LESIONS—71 CASES

Lumbosacral lipoma		
with direct continuation to spinal cord	13	
with direct continuation to filum terminale	3	
without direct internal continuation	2	
	—	18
with diastematomyelia		
without septum, direct continuation to spinal cord	2	
without septum, no connection but bands present	2	
without septum, meningocele manqué	1	
with septum, meningocele manqué	1	
	—	6
Diastematomyelia associated with bands		
without septum	12	
without septum, meningocele manqué	1	
with septum, meningocele manqué	1	
with septum	4	
	—	18
Simple traction by bands		3
Tight filum terminale		5
Lipoma in filum terminale		1
Dermal sinus		1
Coccygeal cyst		2
Meningocele manqué		
true	11	
possible	6	
	—	17
		—
		71

83

the theca. Table 13.1 shows the principal abnormalities of the 71 cases in this group. *Lumbosacral lipomas* are discussed in Chapter 15 and *diastematomyelia* in Chapter 11.

SIMPLE TRACTION BY BANDS

All 3 cases had bands but in 2 of them only the extradural part between a neural arch and the dura mater was found. It is likely that in these 2 cases spinal exploration was inadequate, one was Case 4, very early in our experience, the other, Case 41, provided considerable technical difficulties. Neither has deteriorated subsequently, Case 4 is clinically unchanged and Case 41 has had some improvement in lower limb function and reduction of sensory disturbance. The bands were dense fibrous tissue. One case had hypertrichosis, the other a dimple. The third case (82) in this section had two bands from neural arches Lv5 and Sv1 passing to the conus medullaris at Lv4; both these bands were aberrant dorsal nerve roots as indicated by their sites of origin on the conus medullaris and their histology: there was no external cutaneous manifestation. He was a boy aged $2\frac{1}{2}$ years who presented with ulceration of the toes on one foot, caused by a hot-water bottle. Six years later this leg has absent knee and ankle jerks and no extensor plantar response; there has always been a tendency to hallux valgus and lateral deviation of the toes which has not altered. The other lower limb is normal.

TIGHT FILUM TERMINALE

In the discussion of this condition below, we postulate that tight filum terminale *per se* is not a clinical entity.

There are 14 cases in the whole series in which the filum terminale was tight and had to be divided but most of them were associated with other conditions. The 5 cases shown in Table 13.1 had no associated abnormality beyond local adhesions. In all 5, the filum terminale was clearly tight, it was still strung up in the dorsal part of the vertebral canal after opening of the dura mater and arachnoid and release of cerebrospinal fluid. When divided, the gap between the cut ends in the different cases measured from 1·25 cm to 3·0 cm.

In 2 cases (33, 74) there were no associated adhesions and the conus medullaris (apart from its low situation) and the cauda equina appeared normal. Case 74, a young woman aged 17 years was clinically normal but had hypertrichosis and a very tender naevoid area on the lower back. She continues to be normal 5 years later and she no longer has local tenderness. Case 33 was a boy aged 16 years with trophic ulceration of the toes and anaesthesia of the outer border of the left foot; 6 years later, clinical examination is unchanged but the toes are healed and have had no further ulceration.

In the 3 other cases, the filum terminale was also adherent to the dura mater either laterally or dorsally and remained tight after these adhesions were freed; the possible significance of these adhesions is discussed below with meningocele manqué (p. 96). All 3 cases had unilateral cavovarus. Case 54, a boy aged 4 years, also had diurnal enuresis with very poor control which has recovered to normal in the past 7 years; his foot is unchanged. Case 13 (*Figure 13.1*) a boy aged 9 years with slight hypertrichosis, had cavovarus of one foot with

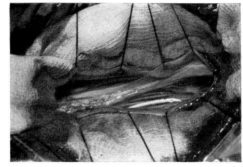

Figure 13.1: Case 13. Dura mater open. The abnormally wide filum terminale is adherent to the dura mater on the right side (Lv5). It is suspended from the dura mater by an arachnoid veil between the point of adhesions and the conus medullaris (Lv3) in the centre of the photograph. (The white object in the lower part of the field is an appearance caused by reflection of light)

Cranial   Caudal

severe inverting spasm which ceased immediately after operation and has not recurred 10 years later; his foot deformity has needed surgical correction. Case 48, a girl aged 13 years with hypertrichosis and a naevoid patch in the lumbar region, has unchanged loss of reflexes and sensation in the foot but the foot deformity has not increased 5 years later and is unlikely to need surgical correction.

Of the remaining 9 cases in which the filum terminale needed division, 3 (26, 38, 53) were associated with lumbosacral lipoma (Chapter 15), 2 (27, 44) with diastematomyelia without septum but with bands (Chapter 11), 3 (10, 56, 100) with meningocele manqué (Chapter 14), and 1 (73) with a lipoma associated with the filum terminale at the end of the dural sac (an atrophied coccygeal cyst, Chapter 13). The gap left between the divided ends measured between 1·0 cm and 3·0 cm. The one with the largest gap (38) was interesting; the filum terminale was associated with a blood vessel which was strung up equally tightly. Leaving the blood vessel intact, the filum terminale was cut and remained suspended by adherence to the blood vessel; the gap between the cut ends was 1·25 cm. After the blood vessel was also divided, the ends of the filum terminale were separated by 3·0 cm.

LIPOMA IN FILUM TERMINALE

Case 81, aged 22½ years, presented with poor circulation, of many years' duration, in both lower limbs, particularly the left which tended to ulcerate above the ankle. The reflexes in the left lower limb were absent and there was absence of sensation in the outer toes. Six years previously a left lumbar sympathectomy had been performed without benefit. At laminectomy the filum terminale was seen to include a lipoma 3 cm long and about 6 cm thick; this part of the filum terminale was excised. The patient was considerably shocked postoperatively but recovered after a few hours. Five years later, there has been no change on neurological examination but there has been no further ulceration.

DISCUSSION

Jones and Love (1956) describe a syndrome associated with tight filum terminale consisting of locomotor difficulties and incoordination of the lower limbs accompanied by pain or numbness, which were most evident on rising from bed in the morning. They describe 6 cases aged between 3 and 35 years, 2 of which had bladder symptoms, but foot deformities were not marked. They account for the early morning onset of symptoms by relating them to the lengthening of the vertebral canal while sleeping in bed, which results from the horizontal position and the increased thickness of the intervertebral discs by water uptake. Only 2 cases had foot deformity—unilateral cavus and claw toes. In 1961, Love, Daly and Harris reported 3 siblings with pes cavus and leg pains and who also had tightness of the filum terminale. They suggested there might be a genetic element because there is such an association in spina bifida cystica. Bilateral idiopathic pes cavus appears to be familial and Schlegel (1964) discusses this aspect in his account of clawfoot associated with spina bifida occulta. He regards the cause as localized in the terminal spinal cord because of the resultant neuromuscular incoordination of the intrinsic muscles of the feet which accounts for the deformity. He postulates that tightness of the filum terminale is the prime factor and advises surgical freeing of the terminal dural sac and division of the filum terminale. Schlegel also quotes Hackenbroch who examined 200 cases of bilateral pes cavus and found lumbosacral laminal defects in 85 per cent; 30 per cent had enuresis as well.

None of our own cases in which the filum terminale appeared to be tight had bilateral pes cavus, nor had any of them the syndrome described by Jones and Love. Numbness of one lower limb was complained of by an occasional patient in our whole series of 100 cases and the absence of complaints of pain was notable in our experience. Bladder symptoms are discussed in Chapter 16.

P.M. Case 137 (Chapter 3) suggests that tightness of the filum terminale by itself does not occur and is therefore not a clinical entity. This case was a chance finding at autopsy; a woman aged 64 who had died following cardiac infarction and who was found to have symptomless diastematomyelia tightly enclosing a bone septum at Lv4 level immediately cranial to the conus medullaris. We have postulated (Chapter 11) that no neurological deficit occurred because the spinal cord was firmly transfixed from early embryonic life and was therefore able to respond by growth with changes in the length of the vertebral canal. If this theory is correct the filum terminale which develops from the neural tube in continuity with the spinal cord (Chapter 2) will also be able to accommodate its growth so there cannot be any such condition as a tight filum terminale. Any success obtained by surgical division of this structure must therefore be due to some other factor which was affected by the operative approach or technique (James and Lassman, 1970). We have 2 cases (p. 84) in which only the filum terminale was divided at operation and there was no other intrathecal abnormality; 1 case had no neurological deficit preoperatively, while the other has unchanged evidence of neuropathy 6 years later although he no longer suffers from trophic ulceration. All the other cases in which the filum terminale was divided had accompanying intrathecal abnormalities as well.

DERMAL SINUS

Other cases of this condition when associated with lumbosacral lipoma have been mentioned (p. 112). The case (55) noted in Table 13.1 was associated with a naevus with which there was no connection and the patient was clinically normal in other respects. Myelography showed no abnormality, the conus medullaris lying at Lv2 level. Dissection showed that the sinus tract passed through a defective neural arch in the lower lumbar region, through the dura and to the conus medullaris at Lv2. There was evidently little traction effect because the conus medullaris was at the adult level and the girl was only 12 months of age. Microscopy showed that the channel was lined by squamous epithelium and became a band with cellular proliferation probably of arachnoid origin and in its deepest part consisted of fat, a small ganglion and a nerve; the intradural part was a nerve.

COCCYGEAL CYST

In Case 73, a boy aged $2\frac{1}{2}$ years, the cyst had existed at birth but atrophied to leave a scarred pigmented naevus and a skin dimple. He had developed a unilateral popliteal palsy which improved considerably in the 5 years after operation and sensation also improved. Survey radiographs showed upper sacral laminal defects but no evidence of sacral agenesis. The only abnormality demonstrated at myelography was the low situation of the conus medullaris—Lv5. At laminectomy an extradural band extended from Sv2 neural arch tissue to the dura mater at Sv1 level but there was no internal continuation. The termination of the dural sac at Sv2 level was occupied by a lipoma surrounding the filum terminale which appeared tight; the filum was cut leaving a gap of 1·5 cm and the lipoma removed.

In contrast, in Case 66, a girl aged 21 months, the coccygeal cyst still existed and at operation was found to be a meningocele extension from the dural sac which extended to the sacrococcygeal joint; the filum terminale was not seen. In all other respects, the child was clinically normal.

Both these cysts were remains of incomplete atrophy of the embryonic tail-bud which should have disappeared during the course of formation of the filum terminale. In Case 73 the dural sac terminated at the normal level but the conus medullaris was situated low down while the cyst had obliterated itself postnatally. In Case 66, the myelogram showed that there was a fine connection between the spinal subarachnoid space and the cyst; the conus medullaris was situated at a slightly lower level than normal.

REFERENCES

James, C. C. M. and Lassman, L. P. (1970). 'Diastematomyelia and the Tight Filum Terminale.' *J. Neurol. Sci.* **10**, 193

Jones, P. H. and Love, J. G. (1956). 'Tight Filum Terminale.' *A.M.A. Archs. Surg.* **73**, 556

Love, J. G., Daly, D. D. and Harris, L. E. (1961). 'Tight Filum Terminale. Report of Condition in Three Siblings.' *J. Am. med. Ass.* **176**, 115

Schlegel, K-F. (1964). 'Spina Bifida Occulta und Klauenhohlfuss.' *Ergebn. Chir. Orthop.* **46**, 268

14—Findings at Operation—IV

TRACTION LESIONS

MENINGOCELE MANQUÉ

Meningocele manqué is a term we have coined for lack of a better expression. In Chapter 15 we refer to 9 cases of atretic meningoceles (p. 110) which are characterized by having a rounded central area of scarred skin, microscopy of material removed from some of them at operation indicating that this was their probable origin. Meningoceles, although the sac itself does not contain functioning neural tissue, commonly have recurrent nerve roots from the spinal cord or cauda equina adherent near the neck of the sac. If the meningocele is very small or if it is well formed at one stage in embryonic or foetal life and then atrophies, it does not necessarily leave any mark on the skin and there may well be nerve roots adherent to the dura mater at the site of origin of the meningeal herniation. At least 11 of our cases were found to have this type of anomaly.

We regard the characteristics of a meningocele manqué as the existence of a loop of recurrent nerve roots or spinal cord tracts which is adherent to the internal surface of the dura mater. Sometimes the adherence is by a single fibrous band, sometimes the loop is held tightly against the dura mater, over a small area, by multiple adhesions. Both types of adherence may be present at the same time and may affect a greater amount of nervous tissue, for example, spinal cord itself, filum terminale and cauda equina, without there being clear evidence of recurrent nerve roots.

It is to be noted that in these cases any discrete band is fibrous. We make this distinction because discrete bands, particularly in association with diastematomyelia, are often aberrant dorsal nerve roots (p. 67). It is true that a band, which would be expected from the operation finding to be a nerve, sometimes proves to be fibrous; in these cases we believe that the aberrant nerve root has failed to

89

find a satisfactory point of contact and consequently cannot function: it therefore atrophies and remains as a strand of fibrous tissue. However, it still is possible in a meningocele sac to find a viable nerve root (*see* Case 96 opposite) so that the histology of the band is not absolute confirmation of the nature of the spinal cord abnormality, but the general rule applies.

Owing to lack of knowledge of the embryology of the lumbar and sacral spinal cord, it is not possible to provide any explanation of the origin of meningocele manqué. Gardner's theory (p. 14) is the only one which bears on the subject.

Table 10.2 shows 11 cases of true meningocele manqué classified on the basis of the findings at operation: 4 had recurrent roots only, 4 adhesions only and 3 had both recurrent roots and adhesions.

Recurrent roots

Case 78 had an atretic meningocele with direct connection to a recurrent root and microscopy of the subcutaneous tissue down to its bone attachment showed appearances similar to that found in the root of a meningocele sac. Five years after laminectomy her clinical condition remains unchanged. She had been born with a mild left talipes equinovarus which had responded well to treatment but started to relapse at the age of 12 years at which time her left plantar response became extensor; in the 6 months before laminectomy her right plantar response also became extensor.

Cases 90 and 93 had no cutaneous abnormality. In both, an extradural band from a spinous process passed through the dura mater to attach at Lv2–3 level to a looped collection of nerves including an ectopic dorsal root ganglion. The band was of fibrous tissue. Both cases presented with early unilateral cavovarus on the same side as the recurrent root had been adherent; in neither case has there been any increase in foot deformity nor any improvement in reflexes in the following 5 years. They were girls aged 3 years and $9\frac{1}{2}$ years at the time of laminectomy.

Case 56, a boy aged 10 years, had a skin dimple which connected to Sv3 spinous process but no deeper attachment was located. The right lamina of Lv5 was inverted and was locally adherent to the dura mater on whose deep surface at this pressure point, the right cauda equina was adherent; it included an ectopic dorsal root ganglion. The nerve roots at this point of attachment were recurrent (*Figure 14.1*). He had presented with a progressive right pes cavovarus and urinary retention with overflow. Five years later he has normal bladder control but the foot deformity needed surgical correction; his abnormal reflexes are unchanged.

Adhesions only

Case 96, a boy aged 14 months, had hypertrichosis and an atretic meningocele which connected directly by multiple adhesions to the conus medullaris and the right cauda equina. The tissue removed at

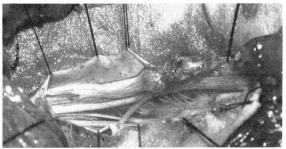

Cranial   Caudal

(a) *Dura mater opened. Right cauda equina is looped and held adherent to dura mater (Lv5); bulbous end of the loop contains an ectopic dorsal root ganglion. A single nerve root from the bulbous loop-end is seen passing obliquely cranially to emerge on the patient's left side*

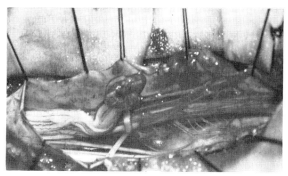

Cranial   Caudal

(b) *After freeing the adherence to the dura mater, the bulbous loop-end lies free. The unusually wide filum terminale can be seen in the centre throughout the length of the open dural sac*

Figure 14.1: Case 56

operation showed on microscopy a small cystic area 5 mm across under the skin and lined by columnar ciliated cells on a thin fibrous base. This cyst lay in the roof of a larger cyst of meningocele origin with a solid fibrous continuation (enclosing a nerve root) which ended in bone. Its further deep extension contained a small nerve and material resembling the filum terminale (the filum terminale was not touched during the operation). Clinically normal at the time of laminectomy, he continues so 5 years later.

In Case 16, the conus medullaris was held to the dorsal dura mater by a fan of dense fibrous adhesions (*Figure 14.2*), in Cases 76 and 77 the cauda equina was bound to the dura mater in the midline. Unilateral spasticity and abnormal reflexes in Cases 16 and 77 have returned to normal 7 and 5 years respectively after laminectomy. (Boy and girl each aged 11 years.) Case 76 has improved bladder control to the extent that he now only suffers from some degree of urgency; his foot deformity has required surgery during the 5 years since laminectomy at the age of 5 years.

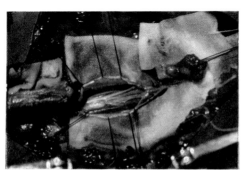

Figure 14.2: Case 16. Dura mater opened. Fatty fibrous tissue in the region of the bifid spine of Lv5 is being held away caudally by a thread. A band is seen extending from it to the dura mater through which it passes to fan out and be attached to the cauda equina and conus medullaris (Lv4)

Cranial   Caudal

Recurrent roots and multiple adhesions

Case 63 had an atretic meningocele but no direct continuation was found. An extradural band held a long loop of the right cauda equina against the internal surface of the dura mater from which there were extensive adhesions binding the conus medullaris and remaining cauda equina to the dura mater. Aged 3 years, the girl had no clinical abnormalities apart from her atretic meningocele, considerable hypertrichosis and multiple laminal defects in the lumbar region. She continues normal 7 years later.

In Case 71, the abnormalities were entirely intrathecal. There was anomalous development of the conus medullaris; the left side being much longer than the right and the cauda equina origins were very irregular. Some of the nerve roots were held up by adhesions to the dura mater and looped back again; all the left cauda equina and the left conus medullaris were also held to the dura over a wide area by dense fibrous tissue. Aged 3 years, this girl presented with hypertrichosis and naevus and was otherwise clinically normal; she continues unchanged 5 years later.

Case 100, a young woman aged 18 years, presented with trophic ulcers and deformity of the left foot. Two years later her foot deformity is unchanged; the trophic ulcers remain healed, but the fifth toe has had to be amputated. The area of sensory loss is very much diminished and is limited to the outer side of the foot and the toes. Her reflexes continued to be absent on that side. At laminectomy, an extradural band was found passing internally to a bundle of nerves of the left cauda equina rolled up in a ball; there were widespread fibrous adhesions to the filum terminale and the remaining roots of the cauda equina (*Figure 14.3*). It was possible to free all these structures.

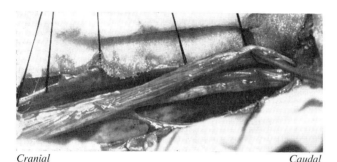

Cranial   *Caudal*

Figure 14.3: Case 100. Loop of recurrent roots of the left cauda equina held by a tough fibrous band to the dorsal dura mater at Sv2 level. The band continued extradurally to the fibrous neural arch of Sv2. The wide filum terminale (4 mm diameter) can be seen at the termination of the dural sac; it had been held dorsally to the recurrent roots by adhesions which had been cleared before this photograph was taken

Possible meningocele manqué

We have placed these 6 cases in this group (*see* Table 10.2) because superficially they resemble the true case. Two had adhesions, in one affecting the conus medullaris (Case 23) and in the other (Case 80) the right cauda equina with similar appearance to *Figure 14.1*. In both, the adhesions also involved a small rounded tumour, light brown in colour, soft but not cystic and in continuity with a nerve. We have regarded these tumours as being ectopic dorsal root ganglions and have encountered them quite frequently. Unfortunately they commonly adhere to neighbouring nerves so that it is not clear whether the local adhesions result from the existence of the ectopic ganglion or whether the fibrosis results from some other process which originally caused the ganglion to be ectopic. The

93

fibrous tissue found in these cases is much less tough than that which we associate with the true meningocele manqué. The remaining 4 cases of possible meningocele manqué had bands connecting the neural arches with intrathecal nervous tissue which was distorted from its normal course. Superficially, therefore, these could well be cases of true meningocele manqué but microscopy showed in each case that

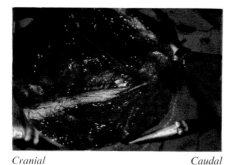

(a) *Extradural band (elevated by probe) passing from the sub-cutaneous tissues (Sv3) to attach to the dura mater*

Cranial　　　　　　　　　*Caudal*

(b) *Dura mater opened. Intra-dural continuation of band; right-hand probe indicates the extradural point of passage (Sv2). The other probe indicates the intrathecal continuation and attachment to the side of the filum terminale. From this point it passes cranially to attach to conus medullaris (Lv4)*

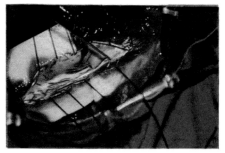

Cranial　　　　　　　　　　　　　*Caudal*

Figure 14.4: Case 10

the band was a nerve. Case 3 had a cutaneous naevus, Case 10 (*Figure 14.4*) a skin dimple but neither Case 42 nor Case 84 had any cutaneous abnormality. In Case 42, besides the band already described there were adhesions of the conus medullaris and filum terminale to the dura mater. In these cases of possible meningocele manqué, our doubts about classification arise because the band in question was a nerve and not tough fibrous tissue (p. 67). However, the material removed in Case 96 (a true meningocele manqué noted above) also contained a nerve, so that possibly the general finding at operation is a better indication of the nature of the origins of the abnormality than the histology of the material removed.

DISCUSSION

From the foregoing, it is clear that meningocele formation by its failure to develop fully or its ability to atrophy once it is formed may well account for an appreciable number of the abnormalities affecting the spinal cord and nerve roots which we have found at operation. We have discussed above 11 cases of true meningocele manqué and a further 6 cases classified as possible; to these we can add a further 14 cases to elaborate our discussion of this subject. The further 14 cases are as follows.

(1) Atretic meningocele (p. 110) Cases 29, 36, 52, 64, 75, 88   6
(2) Lumbosacral lipoma (Table 15.1) with direct continuation to spinal cord. Cases 39, 43   2
With diastematomyelia and septum. Case 72   1
(3) Adherent filum terminale (Table 15.1)
Tight filum terminale. Cases 13, 48, 54   3
Diastematomyelia without septum. Case 27   1
Lumbosacral lipoma, no direct internal continuation. Case 53   1

Cases classified as atretic meningoceles

On page 110, 9 cases of atretic meningocele are noted; 3 of these have been classified as cases of true meningocele manqué and have been discussed above. The remaining 6 cases detailed here had no evidence of direct connection between the skin and the intrathecal structures but it is clear that there was a meningocele at some period earlier in life.

Case 29 had an atretic meningocele in the lower thoracic region which did not come into the laminectomy area Lv1–5, where there was a lumbosacral lipoma. There was nothing to suggest a communication between the naevus and the diastematomyelia with bone septum found at operation. Myelography showed no abnormality apart from the bone septum and the conus medullaris location at Sv1. There were laminal defects Tv8–12 and in the lumbar region. The patient was in other respects clinically normal.

Cases 36 and 88 had diastematomyelia with a bone septum but there was no evidence of connection with the skin naevus and the intrathecal bands were thought to be recurrent roots so were freed and not otherwise interfered with. The skin and subcutaneous tissue from Case 88 had, on microscopy, appearances strongly suggestive of a fibrosed meningocele.

In Case 52 there was a direct connection from the naevus to the dura mater immediately cranial to a bone septum but no internal continuation and the underlying spinal cord appeared normal. The skin and connection to the dura mater were seen on microscopy to contain tissue strongly suggestive of meningeal extension.

Cases 64 and 75 had diastematomyelia without a septum and also a band from extradural tissue passing internally to connection with the filum terminale in the former case and to the spinal cord in the latter. In neither case was any deep connection found from the skin naevus but, again, all the tissues removed at operation suggested, on microscopy, that the densely fibrous intrathecal bands were associated with the meningeal tissue found more superficially. In Case 64 the skin naevus had discharged for a few weeks after birth and had then healed over.

Cases classified as lumbosacral lipomas

The conditions in these cases must also have been of meningocele origin.

Cases 39 and 43 were clearly partial myelomeningoceles but are classified as spina bifida occulta because there was no herniation out of the vertebral canal. Case 39 had an intradural myelocele, the open spinal cord or myelocele rested within the vertebral canal and the open central canal of the spinal cord was plugged with fibrous tissue directly connected to a subcutaneous lipoma (*Figure 15.3*). Case 43 had a kinked spinal cord whose dorsal surface had the same type of connection with the skin. These two cases are gross examples of the type of abnormality occurring in meningocele manqué.

Case 72 is at the opposite extreme from the two cases just cited. Here there was diastematomyelia with a bone septum and there were recurrent tracts adherent to the dura mater. Some of these tracts arose from the spinal cord cranial to the bifurcation and others from the left spinal cord at the diastematomyelia: all returned to near their points of origin. Although there was no traceable connection from the lipoma, there was also an extradural band originating in a neural arch passing internally to attach to the spinal cord cranial to the diastematomyelia; the band was excised and proved to be fibrous and containing a nerve with part of a dorsal root ganglion.

Cases classified as adherent filum terminale

We have discussed the subject of meningocele manqué at length, partly because it gives evidence to explain the origin of some of the extrinsic abnormalities found at operation and also because it enables us to classify a group of cases more explicitly than as cases with the dubious title of 'intrathecal bands and adhesions'. It is likely that we can ascribe the same causation to the 5 cases of adherent filum terminale in all of which this structure was abnormally adherent to the dura mater in such a way as to divert it from its normal central free position amongst the cauda equina. This diversion and the accompanying fibrous adhesions also distorted the course of the conus medullaris which was abnormally rotated in Cases 27 and 53 and the cauda equina on one side in Cases 13, 27 and 54 and on both sides in Cases 48 and 53 (p. 85) (*Figure 13.1*).

Other cases

There is another group of intrathecal adhesions which probably does not fall into the category of meningocele manqué. This group is exemplified by Cases 35, 97 and 101, all of which had diastematomyelia with a septum and the adhesions of the spinal cord to the dura mater could possibly result from previous irritation of traction effects in the same way that when the septum is tightly applied to the caudal bifurcation, the spinal cord is firmly adherent to the arachnoid and dural covering of the septum.

15—Cutaneous Abnormalities on the Back

For ease of expression we have termed these abnormalities external cutaneous manifestations. They can be found in cases without any evidence of neurological deficit or lower limb abnormality and they are not necessarily situated in the locality of an extrinsic lesion of the spinal cord. All the cases in this series had laminal defects but we know that naevi and hypertrichosis can occur without underlying bone defects although we do not know whether spinal cord abnormalities are or are not associated in such cases.

These cutaneous manifestations are of 5 principal types; they may occur singly or in combination, for example, lumbosacral lipoma, hypertrichosis, pigmented naevi, dermal dimples and dermal sinuses. Table 15.1 shows the frequency of these abnormalities amongst our cases.

LUMBOSACRAL LIPOMA

Lumbosacral lipoma is a superficial fatty tumour usually occurring in the lumbar or lumbosacral region in or near the midline (*Figures 15.1, 15.2*). It may be very large and rounded measuring between 20 and 30 cm at the base transversely and rising as much as 15 cm above the surface of the back. We have encountered the largest tumours in younger children while the smaller, being less obvious, are seen in older patients but the excess fat of these smaller swellings is usually distinguishable from normal body fat in moderately obese adults. The very size of the tumour relative to the body of a child causes parents to seek advice so that a number of cases are seen in surgical clinics solely for cosmetic reasons. This is probably why these lipomata are less often seen in adults than children; Flückiger (1967) comments on the different incidence. The less obtrusive lipomas are undetected until neurological deficit occurs and they are then found on routine clinical examination of the back. Analysis of these tumours and their associated cutaneous manifestations is seen in Table 15.2. Lipomatous swellings which are situated mainly to one side of the midline of the back are usually myelomeningoceles.

TABLE 15.1

EXTERNAL MANIFESTATIONS—100 CASES

Lipoma		Naevus	
alone	8	alone	3
with naevus	3	with sinus	1
with naevus and dimple	2		
with naevus and sinus	1	Dimple	
with dimple	2	alone	10
with sinus	2	Sinus	
Hypertrichosis		alone	1
alone	16	Coccygeal arachnoid cyst	1
with lipoma	5	No external cutaneous	
with lipoma and naevus	2	manifestation	27
with lipoma, naevus and dimple	1		
with naevus	14		
with naevus and dimple	1		

TABLE 15.2

LUMBOSACRAL LIPOMAS—26 CASES

ASSOCIATION WITH OTHER CUTANEOUS MANIFESTATIONS

Lipoma		with naevus	3
alone	8	with dimple	2
with hypertrichosis	5	with sinus	2
with hypertrichosis and naevus	2	with naevus and dimple	2
with hypertrichosis, naevus and dimple	1	with naevus and sinus	1

The associated manifestation is usually near either the cranial or the caudal margin of the lipoma. Hair and naevi are commonly cranial and dimples and sinuses caudal, although occasionally the dimple is central.

There are 7 cases with no clinical abnormality, all girls aged between 1 and 10 years, and it is convenient to divide the remaining 19 cases into two groups, Group 1 consisting of 15 children aged 8 months to 12 years, 4 boys and 11 girls, and Group 2—4 adult women aged between 17 and 29 years.

Group 1.—15 Children. Two had a discharging sinus associated with a lipoma; 1 was otherwise clinically normal but the other was incontinent.

Five were affected in both lower limbs, 2 having spasticity, 2 bilateral cavovarus and unilateral limb weakness, and 1 with relapsing club feet and bladder incontinence.

Eight were affected unilaterally. Three were incontinent as well as having whole limb weakness and foot deformity; the other 5 had similar foot deformities associated with paralysis of peronei or of foot invertors or of weakness in these muscles; 1 had a spastic equinus. Most of these cases had sensory loss of some degree including loss of vibration sense and diminished postural sensibility, areas of anaesthesia and of analgesia, and one had trophic ulceration of the toes.

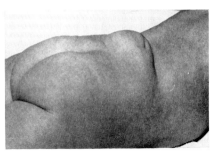

Figure 15.1: Case not in this series. Lumbosacral lipoma with dimple at the apex

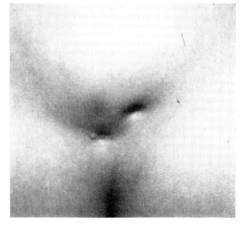

Figure 15.2: Case 15. Lumbo-sacral lipoma with two dimples at the caudal margin

Group 2.—4 Adults. Of these, 2, aged 17 and 23 years, had progressive foot deformity and trophic ulceration which started many years before and had been progressing in a similar pattern to the less severely affected children in Group 1.

Two, aged 25 and 29 years, had no lower limb abnormality but had bladder incontinence, 1 with constant dribbling and the other retention with overflow. Both these patients had been normal until the age of 18 years when they had started developing symptoms of bladder weakness and recurrent infection. This pattern of late onset contrasts with our incontinent cases in Group 1 who seem to have had bladder weakness of varying degree from birth or shortly after.

Brickner (1918) has stated that some cases of lipoma are not

associated with spina bifida but all our cases showed laminal defects
on radiography and widening of the interpedicular distances in the
region of the intrathecal anomaly. Some degree of dysgenesis of the
sacrum existed in 5 patients, 1 of whom had sacral somatoschisis;
none had evidence of bladder weakness in contrast to the cases with
much greater degrees of bone defect (agenesis) reported by Blumel,
Evans and Eggers (1959), Williams and Nixon (1957) and Banta and
Nichols (1969).

TABLE 15.3

RELATIONSHIP OF THE SUBCUTANEOUS LIPOMAS WITH INTRATHECAL
STRUCTURES

DIRECT CONNECTION TRACED—18 CASES

Preoperative State
Normal	3	to spinal cord
Discharging sinus	1	
Discharging sinus and incontinence	1	
Progressive neuropathy	9	
—		14
Normal	1	to filum terminale
Incontinence	2	
—		3
Normal	1	to cauda equina
—		1

NO TRACEABLE CONNECTION—8 CASES

Normal	1	diastematomyelia
Progressive neuropathy	5	
—		6
Normal	1	tight filum terminale
Progressive neuropathy	1	
—		2

Direct traceable connection

Eighteen cases were found to have a direct traceable connection
from the subcutaneous tissues to the spinal cord near or at the conus
medullaris, to the filum terminale or to the cauda equina. These
include all 7 cases with a dimple or sinus except one (53) where the
sinus and lipoma had been previously excised superficially but the
nature of the adhesions around the conus medullaris, filum terminale
and cauda equina suggested that there had previously been a continuity. This case has been classified in Table 15.3 as having a tight
filum terminale because, all the other adhesions having been freed,
the whole terminal nervous tissue fell into more normal relationship

after the filum terminale was cut leaving a substantial gap between its ends. In Case 39, the lipoma stalk attached to the dura mater and continued through it to end by plugging an open intradural myelocele (*Figure 15.3*). The plug was able to be removed; its surface of contact with the spinal cord was lined by ependyma. The spinal cord

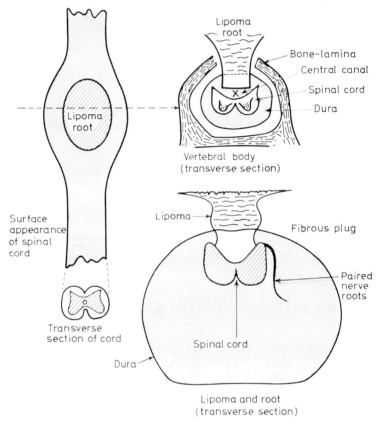

Figure 15.3: Case 39. Lumbosacral lipoma extending intrathecally and plugging an open intradural myelocele (diagrammatic)

rested normally against the vertebral bodies and there was no expansion of the meninges outside the vertebral canal.

There were 7 cases of lipoma without a dimple or sinus which had a similar deep connection. Two of these had had the subcutaneous lipoma removed previously and we do not know whether or not they had dimples originally. It is not possible on our information

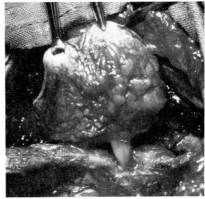

(a) *Case not in this series. Dissection to show lipomatous stalk from lipoma passing between two spinous processes. The muscles have been dissected from the laminae*

Caudal   *Cranial*

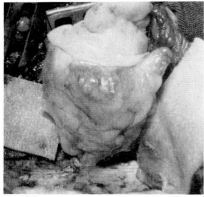

(b) *Case 46. Next stage. Spinous processes and laminae have been removed. Stalk is seen attached to the dura mater*

Caudal   *Cranial*

(c) *Case 46. Dura mater opened. Stalk of the lipoma, drawn to the left, is seen to be continuous with the filum terminale. Compare with Figure 15.10*

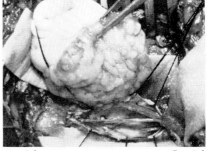

Caudal   *Cranial*

Figure 15.4: Series to show the continuation of a subcutaneous lipoma connecting intrathecally with the intrathecal nervous tissue

103

to state that lipoma cases with dimples are more likely to have a deep connection than those without.

From the nature of the abnormality in this group, neurological deficit is likely to occur at some time in the individual's life, because of increasing tension during growth or by accidental surface movement of the tumour which could then apply a sudden pull upon the nervous tissue (*Figure 15.4*). We have found a similar abnormality in the Manx cat where movement of the tumour caused definite shifting of the spinal cord within the vertebral canal (James, Lassman and Tomlinson, 1969). For reasons unknown, neurological deficit may occur later in life; 2 of these cases developed bladder incontinence at about the age of 18 years and we have another case, not in this series, who became incontinent at the age of 42 years. She fortunately recovered bladder control after spinal exploration at the age of 44 years. A colleague successfully operated on a man aged 26 years who had become incontinent a few years earlier (James and Lassman, 1960, Case A).

No direct traceable connection

Eight cases had no direct traceable connection from the subcutaneous tissues, 6 had diastematomyelia, 3 without a septum but with the bands described in Chapter 13. Although these bands might have been joined to the subcutaneous lipoma no distinct connection was found. The remaining 2 cases had a tight filum terminale.

Superficial analysis of the clinical picture and operation findings (Table 15.3) gives no indication what spinal cord abnormality will be found at operation so a further attempt has been made to discover if there is any correlation. Beyond showing a low-placed conus medullaris, myelography can give no further help in diagnosis.

Clinical picture and operation findings

There is no correlation between the clinical picture and operation findings. Table 15.4 is a modification of Table 15.3.

TABLE 15.4

CONNECTION BETWEEN LIPOMA AND INTRATHECAL STRUCTURES

Traced to		Not traced	8
spinal cord	14		
filum terminale	3		
cauda equina	1		

Taking the 14 cases which had a direct connection to the spinal cord (conus medullaris or immediately adjacent to it) 9 had progressive lower limb neuropathy, 5 had not.

Of the 5 cases without lower limb neuropathy, 3 children were clinically normal, 2 children had a discharging sinus 1 of whom was also incontinent.

Of the 9 cases (including one adult) which had progressive lower limb neuropathy only 2 were affected bilaterally. One (Case 43) had moderate spasticity of both lower limbs and at operation the spinal cord was found to be kinked dorsally and adherent to the dura immediately cranial to the conus medullaris and without herniation from the vertebral canal. The other case (45) had relapsing club feet considered to be clinically significant and was incontinent; she was too young to be accurately tested for sensation. The lipoma connected directly to the conus medullaris.

This leaves 7 cases with unilateral lower limb neuropathy. In 3 there was actual paralysis of foot muscles (peronei or tibiales) while the others had only general muscular weakness of the affected limb. Some had detectable sensory loss, 1 of whom also had trophic ulceration; 1 was incontinent as well. The adult, aged 22 years, had symptoms developing over several years; in early childhood she had been normal. She had increasing weakness of the invertors of one foot, poor circulation, sensory loss and finally trophic ulceration.

In 13 of these 14 cases the conus medullaris was situated at an abnormally low level varying from Lv3 down to Sv2. In the four-teenth case, by contrast, the conus medullaris lay at probably normal level for her age (8 months) over the body of Lv2; she was incontinent and her lower limbs were normal. There was a discharging sinus on the lipoma but the sinus track was blocked just external to its attachment to the dura mater and continued intrathecally as a lipoma (*Figure 15.5*). She had never had meningitis and her operation was not difficult.

In 3 children of the 14 cases being discussed, the filum terminale was not identified and could possibly have been the core of the deep connection; 2 were clinically normal and 1 was affected in one leg and was incontinent. In this context it is interesting to note that the 2 adults who developed bladder incompetence at the age of 18 years and had no lower limb abnormality, had a direct continuation of the subcutaneous lipoma to the filum terminale, that is, the filum termi-nale ended subcutaneously. The conus medullaris was at Lv5 level in 1 and at Sv1 in the other. The only other case with this finding at operation was a clinically normal child aged 5 years whose conus medullaris lay at Lv3 level.

In this correlation, it is not possible to examine the size of the area of attachment to the spinal cord or conus medullaris. There might be a difference between the two types but we have insufficient information. In no case was the site of attachment very large, but of the 2 cases with the largest area of adherence, 1 had bilateral spasticity and was incontinent; and the other, unilaterally affected, became incontinent as a result of the operation owing to the adhesions resulting from previous superficial excision of the lipoma

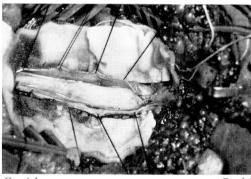

(a) *The dura mater has been opened. The dermal sinus lies to the right held by forceps. The space between the cauda equina is occupied by a lipoma which is a continuation of the dermal sinus and attaches at its other end to the conus medullaris*

Cranial   *Caudal*

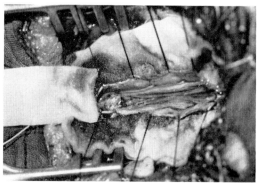

(b) *After removal of the dermal sinus and lipoma. The conus medullaris is seen at the left end of the exposure (Lv2). The lipoma contained ventral horn cells*

Cranial   *Caudal*

Figure 15.5: Case 40

which prevented exploration. In the latter case the full extent of the adherence was not seen at operation while the former case (43) had the spinal cord kinked to be adherent dorsally over a length of about 1·5 cm to the dura within the vertebral canal (almost a myelomeningocele).

Apart from the patients in whom the connection from the lipoma was also the filum terminale, a condition which one might postulate as being potentially liable to produce bladder incompetence, there is no other evidence here to give any indication that a particular abnormality found at operation will be associated with any particular clinical syndrome, and there is no reason to be found why a patient should be incontinent without lower limb neuropathy any more than neuropathy should affect only one limb and not both. Nor is it possible to forecast that a patient at present normal will develop or will not develop a clinical abnormality later in life, but the nature of the surgical findings strongly suggests that a late developing clinical abnormality is likely.

DISCUSSION

In view of this final conclusion we advocate preventive operation on these cases at an early age—about 6 months. We are supported in taking this view by various authors, notably Brickner (1918), Bassett (1950), Dubowitz, Lorber and Zachary (1965), Flückiger (1967) and Loeser and Lewin (1968) and are reinforced in our opinion by the situation of the 2 adults in this series who developed bladder dysfunction at the age of 18 years, our own later adult case aged 44, and Mr. John Hankinson's case which we reported with his permission (James and Lassman, 1960, Case X).

We have so far made little reference to the 7 cases which were clinically normal (Table 15.3) apart from the presence of the subcutaneous lipoma. Their parents wished to have the unsightly prominence removed and their doctors could not be sure that the lipomas were not teratomas or myelomeningoceles. Operations were performed without a prolonged period of observation because preliminary myelography showed an abnormality in every case.

As regards the differential diagnosis there is rarely means of distinguishing the nature of the tumour clinically. A myelomeningocele with a thick layer of subcutaneous fat sometimes does not transilluminate but is more likely to diverge from the midline of the back and myelography is diagnostic. Survey radiographs may show ectopic calcification within the tumour, suggestive of teratoma, but surgery is the final arbiter.

When surgery is undertaken the tumour must be removed and the nervous structures within the dura must be inspected. As our experience has shown, to remove only the tumour without exploring further, makes any further surgery difficult and hazardous. We have 4 such cases in this series including 1 whose original sinus had started to discharge again. All 4 had intrathecal anomalies; 3 of them were satisfactorily treated at operation despite the fibrosis resulting from the previous surgery but in the fourth case it was impossible to expose the spinal cord because the adhesions continued through the dura mater. The operation had to be ended without even an attempt to relieve the tension but unfortunately the child, who had previously been continent, lost her bladder control immediately following the operation. In our whole series of 100 patients reported here and more than a further 50, this is the only patient who has been made worse as a result of operation.

HYPERTRICHOSIS

A hairy patch of skin is commonly associated with spinal dysraph-ism; the most obvious type is that which grows to a considerable

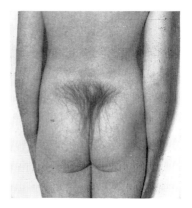

Figure 15.6: Case not in this series.
Hypertrichosis

length resembling a horse's tail (*Figure 15.6*). The patch may be small if situated in the cervical or upper thoracic region of the spine but in the lumbar region where it most commonly occurs it may be extensive laterally. The skin from which the hair grows is often naevoid or pigmented but this may not be seen unless the hair is shaved. Table 15.1 shows the association of hypertrichosis with other cutaneous abnormalities.

There may also be hairy patches where the hair is of a finer silky type, and does not grow so long. It is not difficult to distinguish from an excess of normal hair in the child but, with the full develop-ment of body hair in adult life, it is much less obvious and may be detectable with certainty only if there is some other skin anomaly present. The most common is the naevoid patch.

A third type of hypertrichosis is associated with small pigmented patches of skin in the midline (atretic meningoceles, p. 110) when the hair is sparse and short and is situated around the periphery.

It has been said that hypertrichosis is an indication of underlying diastematomyelia but our cases show that although hypertrichosis is commonly associated with diastematomyelia, it is certainly not indicative. Of 39 cases with hypertrichosis, 20 had diastematomyelia, that is, 51 per cent, whereas of 41 cases of diastematomyelia, 48 per cent had hypertrichosis. Analysis of the 3 types of hypertrichosis mentioned above again shows no definite relationship. Table 15.5 shows the types of spinal cord abnormality associated with hypertrichosis. There is clearly no association of hypertrichosis with any particular spinal cord anomaly.

TABLE 15.5

HYPERTRICHOSIS

CORRELATION WITH OPERATION FINDINGS IN 39 CASES

Hypertrichosis alone		with lipoma, naevus and dimple	
*Diastematomyelia	10	†Traction lesion	1
†Traction lesions	5	with naevus	
Myelodysplasia	1	*Diastematomyelia	6
with lipoma		†Traction lesions	7
*Diastematomyelia	3	Intramedullary dermoid	1
†Traction lesion	1	with naevus and dimple	
Intrathecal myelocele	1	†Traction lesion	1
with lipoma and naevus			
*Diastematomyelia	1		
†Traction lesion	1		

* 20 cases of diastematomyelia: 13 with septum, 6 without, 1 mixed.
† 16 cases of traction lesions: 6 meningocele manqué, 4 tight filum terminale, 4 bands extradural to intrathecal, 2 lipoma pedicle to intrathecal.

Hypertrichosis has occasioned great interest, particularly the horse's tail type because it is such a conspicuous anomaly. Virchow dissected a case of spina bifida occulta because it had a tail and at that time (1875) it was much discussed as evidence of man's descent from tailed ancestry in which context he gave 3 references dated 1812, 1861 and 1669. Von Recklinghausen (1886) in his great work on myelomeningoceles described a case of hypertrichosis in detail. It is possible that Byron, the poet, also had hypertrichosis in which case his foot deformity is accounted for by spinal dysraphism; Lady Caroline Lamb is said to have described him in a letter as 'tailed like a satyr' but her reference may have had a different implication.

PIGMENTED NAEVI

Pigmented naevi are patches which may occur as a single area, rounded and about 5 cm in diameter or much larger near the midline of the back, usually lumbar or lumbosacral. Occasionally there is more than one such area giving the appearance that the original patch has broken into smaller ones around its periphery. The colour varies from bright red to brownish; in some cases patches of one colour shade off into the other giving a mottled appearance; the periphery of such patches is often darker than the more central parts. In one case of thoracic hydromyelia (91) the naevus was over the occiput.

With the exception of one type, termed atretic meningocele, pigmented naevi have no association with any particular spinal cord anomaly.

TABLE 15.6

PIGMENTED NAEVI

CORRELATION WITH OPERATION FINDINGS IN 28 CASES

Naevus alone		with lipoma, hypertrichosis and	
*Diastematomyelia	1	dimple	
†Traction lesion	1	†Traction lesion	1
Hydromyelia	1	with lipoma and dimple	
with hypertrichosis		†Traction lesions	2
*Diastematomyelia	6	with lipoma and sinus	
†Traction lesions	7	†Traction lesion	1
Intramedullary dermoid	1	with sinus	
with lipoma		†Traction lesion	1
*Diastematomyelia	3	with hypertrichosis and dimple	
with lipoma and hypertrichosis		†Traction lesion	1
*Diastematomyelia	1		
†Traction lesion	1		

* 11 cases of diastematomyelia: 6 with septum and 5 without.
† 15 cases of traction lesions: 1 meningocele manqué, 4 tight filum terminale, 6 bands extradural to intradural, 4 lipoma pedicle to intrathecal.

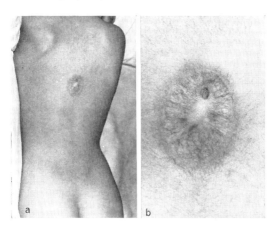

Figure 15.7: Case not in this series. Atretic meningocele. Girl aged 5 years. At birth there was a membranous covering around the edges but the central part was moist. The area slowly granulated over. Laminal defects at Tv9. No clinical abnormality

Atretic meningoceles

Atretic meningoceles (*Figures 15.7, 15.8, 15.9*) constitute 9 of the 28 cases of pigmented naevi analysed in Table 15.6.

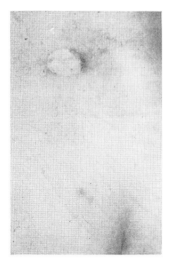 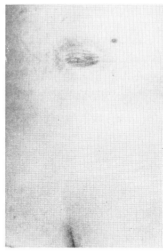

Figure 15.8: Case not in this series. Oval scarred area 1 × ½ inch with slightly raised margin. Slight pigmentation medially. Boy aged 7½ years. At laminectomy no subcutaneous stalk found but there was an extradural band from Lv4 spinous process. There were adhesions on the internal surface of the dura mater with some recurrent nerve roots

Figure 15.9: Case not in this series. Atretic meningocele. Scarred paper-like skin centrally, the peripheral hair has been shaved off. Boy aged 15 months. At laminectomy a fine subcutaneous stalk was found passing through the interspinous area Lv2/3 to the spinal cord at Lv2 level

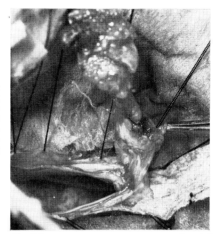

Figure 15.10: Case not in this series. Atretic meningocele with direct continuation to the conus medullaris. The whole tract is shown dissected to its attachment to the conus medullaris (Lv4). The filum terminale was not identified and might have been included in the tract. Compare with Figure 15.4(c)

Caudal   Cranial

111

The skin abnormality is usually rounded, 5 or 6 cm in diameter, and situated in the midline of the lumbosacral area; the central portion is often white and not pigmented, thin with little or no subcutaneous fat and sometimes appears like scar tissue which in fact is probably what it is. The periphery is pigmented, red, pink or brown and often has hair growing out of it—sometimes a silky down, sometimes a horse's tail type of hypertrichosis. These are meningoceles which have atrophied and been absorbed *in utero*; one case (64) was said to have had at birth a small sore at the site which gradually healed over. Microscopy of the skin and deeper tissues confirms this view. The mass beneath the skin commonly contains fibrous tissue which includes structures strongly suggestive of meningeal extension, some clearly associated with small vascular spaces in the manner of arachnoid villi. The extradural part is similar but the intrathecal continuation is commonly densely fibrous.

In 5 cases the direct continuation to spinal cord or cauda equina was easily traced (*Figure 15.10*) but in 1 the direct connection was not found intact extradurally at operation, but the microscopy of the subcutaneous tissues, extradural band and intrathecal continuation demonstrated that they must have been a continuous structure. Of these cases, 3 with direct internal connection also had diastematomyelia, 2 without a septum, the other with a bone septum. All the remaining 3 cases in which no direct continuation to the surface was traced had diastematomyelia with a bone septum. The association of diastematomyelia with myelomeningoceles is well known; it is possible that it is also associated with meningoceles.

The intrathecal extension in some of these cases had similar characteristics to the 'failed meningoceles' which we term meningocele manqué (Chapter 14). The band is fibrous and its attachment to the intrathecal nervous tissue or filum terminale is accompanied by multiple adhesions to the dura. In some cases, the nervous tissue is a loop of recurrent nerve roots or spinal cord tracts held firmly against the dura as is commonly seen in meningoceles. In our meningocele manqué cases, these recurrent roots and fibrous adhesions occur intrathecally usually with an extradural fibrous band connecting to the neural arch area but we commonly fail to find any subcutaneous attachment.

DERMAL DIMPLES AND SINUSES

Dermal dimples

Dermal dimples are skin depressions near the midline with fixation of the epithelium to the underlying layers (Table 15.1) (*Figures 15.11*,

15.12, see also *Figures 15.1, 15.2*). They are not of great importance but they commonly occur on the back in association with spina bifida. Of 16 cases in this series, 4 had a direct traceable continuity,

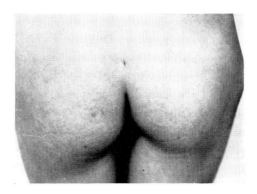

Figure 15.11: Case 11. Sacral dimple

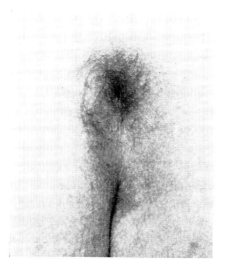

Figure 15.12: Case 25. Sacral dimple with pigmented margins and excess hair

1 to the left spinal cord in diastematomyelia, 1 (containing an intrathecal lipoma) to the filum terminale whose course was distorted, 1 to the conus medullaris and the fourth to attach to recurrent nerve roots. In 3 of these cases the dimple was associated with a lumbosacral lipoma.

The remaining 12 cases had no apparent internal connection; 9

of them were not associated with any other cutaneous abnormality but the remaining 3 were related to lumbosacral lipomas.

Dermal sinuses

Dermal sinuses resemble dermal dimples except that they are much deeper and need to be distinguished from pilonidal sinuses and coccygeal dimples (Table 15.1). The former are regarded as being acquired rather than congenital so are rarely found in children, the latter are situated over the sacrococcygeal area and are of no significance unless they become infected and form abscesses. The dermal sinuses we are referring to are congenital and may be situated at any level of the back; Denis Browne has termed them congenital dermoid sinuses. These sinuses are of considerable importance and potentially dangerous. They may in fact be fistulous, connecting with the subarachnoid space and therefore a common cause of recurrent meningitis. They commonly have ceased to be fistulous having been closed off at laminal or dural level but may still become infected and lead to deep abscesses and meningitis.

In this series we have had 5 cases, 3 of whom had had the subcutaneous part of the sinus excised previously. One of these came to us because he had developed a deep abscess which tracked through the subcutaneous tissues and muscles into the buttock. After drainage of the abscess, its deep surface was explored and a fibrous continuation was located which having penetrated the dura became an intrathecal lipoma and attached to the conus. Subsequent healing was satisfactory and without incident. The second case whose sinus had previously been excised had had two attacks of meningitis; he was referred to us because of later development of paraparesis with incontinence. He had a dermoid cyst with considerable local fibrosis amongst the cauda equina; owing to the adhesions it was only possible to empty the cyst and remove some of its wall. Eight years later he walks well without spasticity but is handicapped by slight contractures of the knees. The third case of this group presented with early cavovarus deformity of one foot and poor bladder control; his conus medullaris, cauda equina and filum terminale were all bound by adhesions to the dorsal dura at Sv1 and the filum terminale was very tight. The adhesions were freed and the filum terminale divided, leaving a substantial gap.

The remaining 2 cases in this group had not been operated on before. In each case the sinus was closed at dural level but continued intrathecally to attach to the conus; in 1 case the continuation was through an intrathecal lipoma which contained non-functioning elements of spinal cord tissue (*Figure 15.5*).

DISCUSSION

Haworth and Zachary (1955) report 18 personal cases of dermal sinuses and dimples and discuss the relation of these abnormalities to pilonidal sinuses. They conclude that the latter are acquired and that the former are congenital, a dimple being a minor form of sinus. They also discuss the nature of these sinuses and agree with Walker and Bucy (1934) that the congenital form results from localized failure of separation of the cutaneous ectoderm from the neural ectoderm during embryological development. They advise exploration and excision of all but very shallow sinuses and dimples because of the risk they carry of permitting the penetration of infection either to cause local abscesses or meningitis. Amador, Hankinson and Bigler (1955) were of the same opinion.

Matson and Jerva (1966) draw attention to sinuses situated in the lumbosacral or coccygeal region which are directed cranially and how important this is in surgical exploration. Since these are embryonic remains, the final skin level of the dermal sinus at birth will be considerably lower on the back than the conus medullaris which has ascended up the vertebral canal in the course of growth and the deep tract will be lengthened accordingly. The sinus tract may become attenuated and stop or it may expand at its inner terminus to form a cystic mass. However, if there is a history of meningitis or if there is any evidence of involvement of the nervous system, the tract is likely to be intact but may be very small and tenuous. They report 8 cases, 7 of which presented with infection and 5 of the latter had had a previous incomplete section of a dermal sinus. Six cases had dermoid cysts and in both the other cases, the tract was followed up to its attachment to the conus medullaris. In all these cases, the surgical exposure to complete the tract excision was considerable. Although myelography will demonstrate the existence of the dermoid cyst, Matson and Jerva insist that the surgical approach should be by way of the sinus and that it should continue until the tract is followed the whole way.

Neither of our cases of dermal sinus had had meningitis but they confirm the statements of Matson and Jerva as regards the cranial direction of the tracts, both of which had attenuated at dural level but could be followed intrathecally.

A recent case of ours had a sinus which was related to a subcutaneous dermoid cyst; at the age of 4 years, the tract and cyst were excised superficially elsewhere but because of renewed symptoms further exploration at the age of 17 years revealed a continuation of the sinus tract through a spinous process to end at the dura. However, on opening the theca, a lump of dermoid caseous material was found lying loose in the subarachnoid space; owing to the blockage of the subcutaneous end of the tract, the debris from the tract had evidently leaked intrathecally. There was no history of meningitis.

REFERENCES

Amador, L. V., Hankinson, J. and Bigler, J. A. (1955). 'Congenital Spinal Dermal Sinuses.' *J. Pediat.* **47**, 300

Banta, J. V. and Nichols, O. (1969). 'Sacral Agenesis.' *J. Bone Jt. Surg.* **51A**, 693

Bassett, R. C. (1950). 'The Neurological Deficit Associated with Lipomas of the Cauda Equina.' *Ann. Surg.* **131**, 109

Blumel, J., Evans, E. B. and Eggers, G. W. N. (1959). 'Partial and Complete Agenesis or Malformation of the Sacrum with Associated Anomalies.' *J. Bone Jt. Surg.* **41A**, 497

Brickner, W. M. (1918). 'Spina Bifida Occulta.' *Am. J. med. Sci.* **155**, 473

Dubowitz, V., Lorber, J. and Zachary, R. B. (1965). 'Lipoma of the Cauda Equina.' *Archs. Dis. Childh.* **40**, 207

Flückiger, A. (1967). 'Les Tumeurs Lombosacrées associées au Spina Bifida Occulta.' *Archs. suisses Neurol. Neurochir. Psychiat.* **99**, 201

Haworth, J. C. and Zachary, R. B. (1955). 'Congenital Dermal Sinuses in Children. Their Relation to Pilonidal Sinuses.' *Lancet* **2**, 10

James, C. C. M. and Lassman, L. P. (1960). 'Spinal Dysraphism. An Orthopaedic Syndrome in Children Accompanying Occult Forms.' *Archs. Dis. Childh.* **35**, 315

— — and Tomlinson, B. E. (1969). 'Congenital Anomalies of the Lower Spine and Spinal Cord in Manx Cats.' *J. Path. Bact.* **97**, 269

Lassman, L. P. and James, C. C. M. (1967). 'Lumbosacral Lipomas: Critical Survey of 26 Cases Submitted to Laminectomy.' *J. Neurol. Neurosurg. Psychiat.* **30**, 174

Loeser, J. D. and Lewin, R. J. (1968). 'Lumbosacral Lipoma in the Adult.' *J. Neurosurg.* **29**, 405

Matson, D. D. and Jerva, M. J. (1966). 'Recurrent Meningitis Associated with Congenital Lumbosacral Dermal Sinus Tract.' *J. Neurosurg.* **25**, 288

Recklinghausen, F. von (1886). 'Untersuchungen über Spina Bifida.' *Virchows Arch. Path Anat. Physiol.* **105**, 243–330; 373–455

Virchow, R. (1875). *Verh. berl. Ges. Anthrop. Ethnol. Urgesch.* 279. (supplement in *Z. Ethnol.* 1876. 7)

Walker, A. E. and Bucy, P. C. (1934). 'Congenital Dermal Sinuses: A Source of Spinal Meningeal Infection and Subdural Abscesses.' *Brain* **57**, 401

Williams, D. I. and Nixon, H. H. (1957). 'Agenesis of the Sacrum.' *Surgery Gynec. Obstet.* **105**, 84

16—Incontinence

By incontinence we mean lack of bladder control. Since few of our patients were examined by a urologist before we operated on them, we have no detailed information about their disability apart from the symptomatology. Our patients could be classified into two groups, those suffering from total incontinence and those with sphincter weakness.

Total incontinence.—There is a continual leak of urine. Since we have no information about the presence or absence of bladder distention, this group probably includes cases with retention and overflow. We had 18 cases including 4 adults.

Sphincter weakness.—The patient is commonly dry in bed at night and has periodic involuntary emptying of the bladder in the day-time particularly on standing out of bed in the morning. Bladder sensation is often present. There were 6 cases.

With all types of incontinence, the older patient has usually learnt to minimize the embarrassment of involuntary wetting by regular bladder emptying or by remaining close to toilet facilities whenever possible.

Of the 24 patients in the whole group, 14 had incontinence of some kind as the principal reason for our investigating them. In the remaining 10 cases, the urinary disabilities were a secondary consideration (paraplegia or paraparesis in the majority) although 8 were totally incontinent and 2 had sphincter weakness.

A minor degree of sacral dysgenesis existed in 3 cases, 2 with sphincter weakness and 1 with total incontinence.

Table 16.1 lists the abnormalities found at operation and, as with most of the 100 cases in our series, they were all sited in the lumbo-sacral spinal cord or had an effect upon it by traction. All 5 cases of dermoid cyst (in the whole series) are in this group of cases, otherwise the list does not indicate any particular abnormality as a cause for incontinence.

117

Many years ago, it was suggested that a tight filum terminale caused incontinence but because cutting this structure failed to cure nocturnal enuresis the idea fell into disrepute. From our observations in the clinic we had at one time gained the impression that the

TABLE 16.1

INCONTINENCE: OPERATION FINDINGS IN 24 CASES

Spinal cord compression by transverse dural band		1
Myelodysplasia		1
Intrathecal bands, adhesions and recurrent nerve roots		2
Diastematomyelia, with aberrant roots and adhesions		5
Lumbosacral lipoma		
with filum terminale as direct continuation	2	
with direct continuation to spinal cord	3	
	—	5
Dermal sinus to conus medullaris		1
Dermoid cysts		
in spinal cord	3	
in cauda equina	2	
	—	5
Filum terminale tight and needing division		
Extradural band to spinal cord	1	
Adhesion of filum terminale to dura mater	1	
Recurrent nerve roots	1	
Lumbosacral lipoma without deep connection	1	
	—	4
		24

original suggestion might have some substance and we have mentioned the subject again in our section on lumbosacral lipomas (Chapter 15). However, careful examination of all our information provides us with nothing to substantiate the idea. That there might be no such clinical entity as a tight filum terminale (Chapter 13) had not at that time suggested itself to us. A tight filum terminale implies traction on the spinal cord; we therefore reviewed our operation findings from this point of view so that we could compare those who had incontinence with those who did not. In both groups there were abnormalities which might produce traction on the conus medullaris or caudal spinal cord but the symptomatology was so varied that we were unable to formulate any correlation. We also compared the operation findings in cases with incontinence with the clinical results (Table 16.2) and again could find no correlation. Therefore we can neither say that there is any particular abnormality which is likely to cause incontinence nor can we say which kind of abnormality will respond to surgical correction and so give an expectation of controlling the incontinence.

There is one factor which we cannot examine satisfactorily and that is the result of operation relative to the preceding duration of incontinence or the age of onset. The history of incontinence of any kind in a small child is difficult to obtain; with quite a number of our patients, the parents were unaware that there might be any physical

TABLE 16.2

INCONTINENCE—24 CASES

RESULTS COMPARED WITH OPERATION FINDING

Case No.	Type of incontinence	Age at operation	Operation finding
NORMAL			
18	Total	28 years	Lumbosacral lipoma to filum
62	Total	18 months	Myelodysplasia
70	Total	$2\frac{1}{2}$ years	Dermoid cyst in spinal cord
56	Total	$10\frac{1}{4}$ years	Recurrent nerve roots
88	Total	$9\frac{1}{2}$ years	Diastematomyelia etc.
10	Sphincter weakness	6 years	Tight filum terminale
54	Sphincter weakness	$4\frac{1}{2}$ years	
45	Sphincter weakness	16 months	Lumbosacral lipoma
IMPROVED			
2	Total	$4\frac{1}{2}$ years	Spinal cord compression by dural bands
23	Total	3 years	Intrathecal bands, adhesions etc.
75	Total	19 years	Diastematomyelia etc.
25	Total	25 years	Lumbosacral lipoma to filum
76	Total	5 years	Intrathecal bands, adhesions etc.
83	Total	9 years	Diastematomyelia etc.
86	Total	22 months	
79	Sphincter weakness	$9\frac{1}{2}$ years	Lumbosacral lipoma
UNCHANGED			
19	Total	$2\frac{1}{4}$ years	Lumbosacral lipoma
40	Total	8 months	Dermal sinus
95	Total	44 years	Dermoid cyst in spinal cord
99	Total	$3\frac{1}{2}$ years	
67	Total	9 years	Dermoid cyst in cauda equina
31	Total	8 years	
60	Sphincter weakness	6 years	Diastematomyelia etc.
53	Sphincter weakness	$10\frac{1}{2}$ years	Tight filum terminale

reason for the child's lack of control. One of our patients was a boy aged 10 years who was referred because of progressive foot deformity together with the statement that there was no bowel or bladder disturbance: the parents and family doctor had thought that the boy's retention with overflow was a behaviour problem but it was genuinely neurogenic. With the 4 adults aged 28, 25, 44 and 19 years, we know that onset of incontinence was respectively at the ages of 18 years, 18 years, 38 years and very early childhood. Whereas the patient aged 44 years had had two operations to correct her incontinence, the other 3 patients had had no treatment.

When considering improvement in bladder control in children, without specific renal tract investigation before laminectomy, any subsequent recovery of control can be ascribed to growing-up and to training. For example Case 62, a boy aged 18 months at time of operation, has gradually recovered complete control during the ensuing 7 years, although the operation finding of myelodysplasia was untreatable (p. 80). In Case 23, we had not thought at the time of operation that we had been able to benefit the child; she had intrathecal bands and adhesions which would not appear to be causing any trouble. However, between the ages of 3 years at operation, when she was totally incontinent, and 10 years, she has developed a considerable degree of bladder control; her anal reflex is present on the right side but absent on the left.

Case 18 illustrates the importance of early diagnosis; aged 28 years at the time of laminectomy, she was totally incontinent and had a history of progressive urinary difficulty and infection since she was 18 years of age. Three months after laminectomy she had regained normal bladder control but subsequently she developed ascending pyelitis and hydronephrosis necessitating ureteric diversion and cystectomy.

Bowel incontinence has not been a feature amongst these cases except as chronic constipation and unfortunately the state of the anal reflex has not been recorded in many cases. Where it has been noted, the state of the anal reflex is as follows (the case numbers can be associated with the operation findings and results in Table 16.2).

Absent before operation, now present   Case 25
Absent before operation, unchanged   Cases 18, 67, 79, 95
Present before operation, unchanged   Cases 56, 62, 83, 88
Previously not recorded, now absent   Cases 19, 75
Previously not recorded, now present   Cases 2, 10, 31, 53, 54, 70, 86

In Case 23 previously not recorded, left reflex absent, right present.

Review of the literature on this subject has not been very enlightening. The term enuresis without qualification is commonly used for almost every form of urinary complaint and our own classification is little more specific.

17—Congenital Foot Abnormalities

Table 17.1 sets out the details of 18 cases, 2 of which can be excluded because of the ambiguity of the birth history. The boy with the weaker leg (Case 91) later developed a paralytic foot-drop, and spinal weakness; laminectomy at the age of $1\frac{1}{2}$ years showed extensive hydromyelia from Cv5 to Tv8. The other child (Case 11) came to operation at the age of $12\frac{1}{2}$ years because of cavovarus of the same foot on which her fifth toe was said to be enlarged at birth; she also had sensory and reflex loss. Laminectomy showed an intrinsic transverse thickening in the dura mater, the fibres being oblique and much thicker at its caudal edge; this transverse band was compressing the intrathecal contents at the level of the lumbosacral joint well below the conus medullaris, the cauda equina could be the only structure compressed and yet the neurological deficit was strictly unilateral. This finding can only be described as ambiguous and has been classified as negative but the plantar reflex and knee jerk have subsequently recovered to normal; the ankle jerk is still absent and the sensory loss unchanged.

The congenital foot deformity in the remaining 16 cases could not have been diagnosed at birth as being neurogenic although it could have been suspected in Case 60. At the age of 12 months, 3 of them with talipes equinovarus manifestly had neurological deficit; 2 bilateral cases (62, 45) had early paraplegia and the other (58) unilateral spastic equinovarus. At the age of 2 years, Case 72 with unilateral talipes calcaneovalgus developed a sore toe and was found to have abnormal reflexes; Case 99, with unilateral talipes equinovarus, developed paraplegia. The remaining cases developed their neurological deficits when aged between 4 and 17 years.

There were 14 cases of talipes equinovarus, 4 of them bilateral of whom 3 developed paraplegia. One unilateral case (99) also became paraplegic. One unilateral case (60) had a vertical talus in the other foot and was incontinent; she had diastematomyelia without a septum and there was no cutaneous manifestation. At operation, 9 of them had diastematomyelia, 2 had meningocele manqué, 1 had myelodysplasia, 1 had an intramedullary dermoid and 1 had a lumbosacral lipoma connecting to the spinal cord. In this group,

TABLE 17.1

CONGENITAL FOOT ABNORMALITIES—18 CASES

Talipes equinovarus	
Unilateral, progressing to abnormal reflexes and sensory loss	3
progressing to ulceration	5
progressing to paraplegia	1
with incontinence and other foot vertical talus	1
Bilateral, progressing to abnormal reflexes and sensory loss	1
progressing to paraplegia	3
	14
Talipes calcaneovalgus	
Unilateral, progressing to abnormal reflexes and sensory loss	1
Foot-drop	
Unilateral progressing to ulceration	1
Ambiguous birth history	
Enlargement of fifth toe	1
Left leg and foot weaker than right	1

apart from a rather high proportion of cases of diastematomyelia there is no real relation between the operation findings and unilaterality or bilaterality nor is there any association with the clinical syndrome.

Of the remaining 2 cases, 1 had unilateral talipes calcaneovalgus with neurological deficit and diastematomyelia, and the other (Case 14) unilateral foot-drop at birth which slowly recovered but she gradually developed a varus foot with subsequent paretic valgus, lateral deviation of the toes, hallux valgus and sensory loss: at operation at the age of 6 years she also was found to have diastematomyelia.

18—Adults

Of the 100 cases reviewed here, 12 were adults aged 16 to 44 years, 2 male and 10 female. They presented in two groups, 3 females with incontinence aged 25, 28 and 44 (Cases 25, 18, 95) who are included in the discussions on pages 100, 120 and Chapter 12, and the remaining 9 because of lower limb abnormalities. In the first group the symptoms were of only a few years' duration, in the second group the onset of symptoms with one exception (Case 74) had been in childhood. Cases 33 and 84, aged 16 years and 18 years respectively, had had symptoms starting at about 15 years of age while the other cases had started very much younger. The syndromes occurring were similar in all respects to those in the children in this series and it is surprising that foot deformities and trophic ulceration had been tolerated for so long.

The exceptional case (74) aged 17 years was clinically normal but presented with hypertrichosis and a painful naevus; she is discussed on p. 84. Case 75, a male aged 19, presented with recent foot-drop but had always had defective bladder control.

There are relatively few adults in this series because the association of spina bifida occulta with incontinence and foot deformity is not well known. We see a certain number of cases attending the out-patients' department for the supply of surgical footwear and calipers. These patients almost always ascribe their abnormalities to the effects of poliomyelitis in childhood or to hypothetical injuries in infancy, even those who have had toes amputated because of recurrent sepsis. One patient had had a below-knee amputation of one leg. We have not investigated these patients, apart from survey radiography, because the spinal cord injury must be irreversible owing to its long duration so that laminectomy is unlikely to benefit. Myelography would be of considerable but academic interest and is not justifiable. In some cases, onset of clinical abnormality occurs after childhood and if diagnosis were possible shortly after onset, myelography and laminectomy would be worth while. We saw one patient aged 56 years with tetraplegia of 15 years' duration; we found at myelography that she had diastematomyelia with a septum at C4–5 level. The question of operation was discussed and refused; we had not pressed the matter because of our doubt about the wisdom of a major surgical procedure in one so frail and with equivocal chances of success. In this particular instance, it is difficult to explain why this anomaly should give trouble so late in life. This is the only case of diastematomyelia with septum in the cervical spine that we have seen.

Our experience suggests that the commonest first symptom of spina bifida occulta occurring in adult life is incontinence. Most of our cases are women; we have reported 3 cases here and have had other cases with symptoms starting in the fifth decade of life. These have been operated on successfully but our oldest patient, a man of 66 years with urinary (non-prostate) symptoms starting about 2 years ealier, was not relieved by laminectomy although there were significant findings at operation. Diastematomyelia producing first symptoms in adult life is reported by English and Maltby (1967) who describe 2 cases presenting with lower limb neuropathy and refer to 5 other reported cases. Freeman (1961) reports another. The symptoms in these cases first occurred between the ages of 32 and 48 years. Our case, a woman aged 64 years, shows that diastematomyelia found at autopsy (p. 22), with a bone septum situated even as low as Lv4 does not always cause damage.

We have not come to any decision as to when a patient is too old to be operated on. The decision will depend on the patient's general physical condition and the duration of symptoms, possibly also their severity.

REFERENCES

English, W. J. and Maltby, G. L. (1967). 'Diastematomyelia in Adults.' *J. Neurosurg.* **27**, 260

Freeman, L. W. (1961). 'Late Symptoms from Diastematomyelia.' *J. Neurosurg.* **18**, 538

19—Results after Laminectomy

In selecting cases for laminectomy, we have laid down three criteria without which a surgically treatable abnormality is unlikely to be found. There must be (1) abnormality of gait and deformity of the foot, unilateral or bilateral, which is either progressive associated with neurological deficit or there is neurogenic incontinence; (2) radiographic evidence of laminal defects of a greater degree than only of Sv1; and (3) myelographic evidence of abnormality or a low-placed conus medullaris.

There are two exceptional types of case outside these criteria: those with a discharging sinus or fistula on the back because they run the risk of recurrent meningitis, and those cases with a lumbo-sacral lipomatous swelling, the majority of which have a direct connection from the subcutaneous tissues to the spinal cord (Chapter 15). We believe that the second group of cases should be operated on as a preventive measure provided that the operation includes an exploration of the spinal cord at the same time as the removal of the lipoma. The lipoma must not be removed superficially without this deep exploration.

All the cases in this series were operated on more than 5 years ago. One case (29) was killed in a road accident 18 months after operation; she was clinically normal at the time of operation apart from a lumbosacral lipoma and was still normal when examined 1 year later; she had diastematomyelia with a bone septum. Seven cases have failed to attend for recent review; 3 were seen 2 years after operation, 1 unchanged, 1 possibly improved and 1 improved at that time; 2 were seen 3 years after operation, 1 still normal and 1 unchanged; 2 were seen 4 years after operation, both improved. The remaining 92 cases have been followed up for between 5 and 13 years (Table 19.1).

The purpose of spinal exploration is to remove any extrinsic abnormalities which affect the spinal cord or nerve roots so that there will be no further neurological deterioration. Our results show that we have achieved this rather negative object but give no indication of which type of case is likely to benefit by spinal exploration. One improvement which has occurred in some cases and which we cannot explain is the rapid healing of trophic ulceration postoperatively in spite of continued sensory loss (*Figure 19.1*). Ulcers do not recur where there are no foot deformities or if the deformities have been corrected; they will recur if there is residual deep infection and if the foot deformity is such that weight is not borne correctly or the shoes do not fit. We have also noted improvement in the appearance of skin circulation and a few patients have commented on the subjective improvement in limb warmth which is occasionally quite definite on palpation. The first evidence of improvement is commonly seen within 3 months after laminectomy but improvement in bladder control may take 2 years.

TABLE 19.1

RESULTS AND LENGTH OF FOLLOW-UP

	Years 1–4	5–6	7–9	10–13	Total
Normal	2	5	8	2	17
Worse	0	0	1	1	2
Unchanged	2	21	10	5	38
Unchanged/improved	1	1	7	0	9
Improved	3	11	12	8	34
Total	8	38	38	16	100

In what follows, the surgical finding 'tight filum terminale' is used for the sake of simplicity. This term includes a variety of abnormalities of this structure and reference should be made to Chapter 13 for more detailed information.

NORMAL BEFORE AND AFTER OPERATION (17 CASES)

The cases which were normal before surgery and continued to be normal after operation had external cutaneous manifestations; 7 with lumbosacral lipoma, 7 with hypertrichosis, 1 with a coccygeal cyst and 2 with dermal sinuses. The two last named cases were not classified as normal in Table 10.1. The operation findings in these cases were as follows.

Lumbosacral lipomas

In 4 the lipoma connected directly through to the intrathecal

126

neural tissues and in a further case the direct connection plugged the gap between the 2 spinal cords of diastematomyelia. One case had diastematomyelia with a septum and 1 had a tight filum terminale.

Hypertrichosis
Three had diastematomyelia with a septum, 1 had partial dia-stematomyelia with adhesions; 2 had meningocele manqué and 1 a tight filum terminale.

Coccygeal cyst
The case with a coccygeal cyst had a meningocele connecting with the main subarachnoid space.

Sinus
The 2 cases with a sinus had a direct connection through to the neural tissue but the sinus was obliterated at the point of penetration of the dura.

WORSE (2 CASES)

Case 19 was operated on at the age of $2\frac{1}{2}$ years because she was incontinent, probably from birth, but otherwise had no neurological deficit. She had a lumbosacral lipoma which had a direct continuation down to the conus medullaris at Sv2 level. The filum terminale was not definable. For $4\frac{1}{2}$ years afterwards, her physical state and incontinence were unchanged but then a cavovarus foot action started to develop and she gradually became paraplegic during the next 2 years. She was able to walk about without any support but rather clumsily; her left foot deformity increased so that she required heel cord elongation and bone correction of the mid-tarsal region. Following this her gait improved considerably and when last seen, 10 years after laminectomy, the state of paraplegia was slight. Originally her myelogram had shown a low conus with an oval filling-defect posteriorly at Sv1–3; this was the area which was explored.

Case 49 is the only case in our series which has been made worse by the operation itself. This was a girl aged 6 years who had had a lumbosacral lipoma removed for cosmetic reasons some years earlier. She was referred to us because the orthopaedic syndrome, which we have described, had started in one foot with sensory loss. At lamin-ectomy we found that the fibrosis ensuing from the previous opera-tion was very extensive and that the dura mater was so firmly adherent to the spinal cord and nerve roots that it was not possible to do anything; the operation was promptly terminated. Immediately after this she became incontinent with loss of her anal reflex, which has not recovered during the 7 years that she has been followed. Her cavovarus deformity has slowly increased and the foot has had to be operated on to make it plantigrade. Her orthopaedic condition is now static.

UNCHANGED (38 CASES)

Our negative object in preventing further deterioration by surgical exploration would appear to have been successful. By the nature of the operation findings, it is evident that some cases would have become worse if left untreated but equally there are probably a number of cases which would not have become worse if left alone. From the clinical standpoint we continue to be unable to distinguish which cases will benefit and which will not. An established foot deformity in a child will continue to grow worse during the remaining growth period even when the primary cause has been removed; it is therefore difficult to know whether spinal exploration has been successful or not, particularly because sensory loss is so very difficult to assess in the very young.

In 23 cases, the normal anatomy of the spinal cord and nerve roots was sufficiently distorted by bands and adhesions or by pressure by a septum in diastematomyelia that it is almost certain that freeing of these structures benefited the patients. Six cases had a lumbosacral lipoma with direct continuation to the neural structures; 3 of these were incontinent, 2 had unilateral foot deformity and 1 had paraplegia. One case with mild foot deformity and abnormal reflexes had a very tight and laterally adherent filum terminale. Four cases had adhesions and bands of meningocele manqué type; they all had unilateral foot deformity. Two cases had dermoid cysts; both were incontinent and had paraparesis. Nine cases had diastematomyelia, 5 with a septum, 4 without; all of them had unilateral foot deformity. The last case in this group was a woman aged 22 with foot deformity; the filum terminale contained a fibro-lipoma which was excised.

In 15 cases, the operation findings were such that either there was nothing capable of surgical remedy or it was impossible to determine how the bands or septum could affect the neural structures. In the first group there were 5 cases, 1 with a thickened enlarged conus medullaris (myelodysplasia), 1 with diastematomyelia without a septum and without bands, 2 with extradural bands which had no traceable intradural continuations and 1 case with a localized

thickening of the dura mater without evidence of intrathecal abnormality. All these cases presented with unilateral deformity and
abnormal reflexes. In the second group of 10 cases, the intrathecal
bands, adhesions or septa found at operation did not appear to have
any real distorting effect upon the neural structures; 9 of them had
unilateral foot defects (including 1 with incontinence also) and 1 had
had a tender naevus on her back and abnormal reflexes.

In this latter group, Case 86 is notable because she had two separate
laminectomies, the first when aged 1 year 10 months because of
increasing inversion activity of her insensitive right foot, urinary
incontinence and severe constipation. Myelography showed extensive diastematomyelia with probable septa at Tv9, Tv11 and Lv5
levels so the lumbosacral area was explored. A partly ossified septum
was found passing obliquely from the pedicle/laminal area to the
midline of the vertebral body; when it was removed there was no
evidence of compression of the right spinal cord but this was only
half the diameter of the left spinal cord throughout the area which
could be examined from Lv3 level down to where the two spinal
cords joined to form the conus medullaris immediately caudal to the
septum. No cranial junction of the two spinal cords was visible
cranially but there were a number of commissural bands between
them. During the next 4 years, there was no change clinically but she
developed a chronic trophic ulcer under the head of her right first
metatarsal and the foot and leg were cyanotic. There had been
improvement in bladder control but constipation continued and there
had been no change in the area of sensory loss in the right foot.
The left lower limb was normal as it had always been. Myelography
confirmed the previous findings in the lower thoracic region and
laminectomy in the area Tv6–11 was done when she was $6\frac{1}{2}$ years old.
There was a partly ossified septum at Tv9 and commissural bands at
Tv11 level; there was also an aberrant nerve root from the left
spinal cord which penetrated the septum and was removed when the
septum was taken away. The two spinal cords in this area were of
equal size and joined together at Tv6 level but there was no evidence
of junction, so far as could be seen, down to Tv12. Postoperatively
the only significant change was subjective and objective improvement
in the warmth and circulation of the right leg. The trophic ulceration
healed slowly but recurred and persisted owing to fixed foot deformity and absence of sensation; a Syme's amputation was performed when she was 8 years old by which age she had much better
urinary control but suffered from recurrent mild cystitis. At the time
of her first laminectomy, the possibility was considered that release
of the spinal cord in the lumbar region might later produce symptoms

from pressure of the thoracic septum but at the second laminectomy it was clearly not causing any undue pressure and there was no obvious cause for interference with spinal cord function unless the existence of an aberrant nerve root passing to the septum was responsible.

UNCHANGED, POSSIBLY IMPROVED (9 CASES)

The assessment of improvement is based on the patient's own subjective sensation or on our own, possibly biassed, opinion. In some cases the improvement could be due to normal growth and development.

Case 27 had early cavovarus gait with some weakness in the right foot. Her knee and ankle jerks were absent. Originally there was some sensory loss in the foot but 9 years later there is no detectable loss of sensation, the knee jerk is present and there has been no deterioration in her foot shape, although the heel cord has had to be lengthened. Aged 3 years at the time of operation, she had diastematomyelia without a septum and no bands; the conus medullaris and the filum terminale were rotated and adherent laterally to the right dura. The adhesions were divided and the filum terminale cut.

Case 28, aged $10\frac{1}{2}$ years, had a cavovarus deformity of one foot with ulceration of the great toe. Her reflexes and sensory loss remain unchanged but there has been no further ulceration. We have had a number of cases which have not had further ulceration; the operation seems to be able to improve the action of the sympathetic nerve supply without changing sensation. This child's foot deformity has required surgical correction. The case has been followed for $7\frac{1}{2}$ years. She had diastematomyelia with a fibrous septum which was not causing any pressure. The laminae in the area of the diastematomyelia were inverted and causing pressure.

Case 33, a boy aged 16 years at time of laminectomy, had symptoms (similar to Case 28) starting about 12 months previously; his toe sepsis has healed and remained healed, but he still has sensory loss in them. He has not had subjective sensory improvement. The clawing of his toes remains slight and he is likely to be able to continue like this permanently without orthopaedic operations. The case has been followed for 6 years. He had a tight filum terminale which on division left a gap of 1·25 cm.

Case 34, aged $17\frac{1}{2}$ years at operation, had a long history of clawed toes and chronic sepsis which did not improve after laminectomy but she recovered subjective sensation with a feeling of warmth in the left foot. There was slight improvement in the area of sensory loss but recurrent sepsis in a deformed foot necessitated below-knee amputation 7 years postoperatively. She had an extensive diastematomyelia without septum with two bands passing from a subcutaneous lipoma to attach to the spinal cord. The traction by the bands made the left spinal cord tend to overlap the right one.

Case 42 presented at the age of 9 years with a cavovarus gait and some sensory loss. Her area of sensory loss is reduced and although she still has mild pes cavus, her gait is normal. There is also subjective sensory improvement 8 years postoperatively. She had a band from Lv4/5 neural arch passing through the dura to attach to the conus. There were also adhesions of the conus medullaris and the filum terminale fixing them to the dura dorsally; these were freed.

Case 53 presented with early right foot deformity, some hyperalgesia in the affected foot and urinary sphincter weakness. He was aged 10 years and in early infancy had had a lipoma with discharging sinus excised from the lumbosacral region. He did not attend for follow-up review for 4 years because he joined the merchant navy. His foot deformity ceased to increase and he has recovered control of his bladder during the followed-up of 7 years. At laminectomy, his conus medullaris, filum terminale and cauda equina were all adherent to the fibrous arch of Sv2. When the adhesions had been divided and the filum terminale cut, there was no tension on any of the neural structures.

Case 58, aged 16 months at the time of laminectomy, presented with equinovarus spasticity of the left foot. At operation she was found to have diastematomyelia with a bone septum causing considerable pressure at the bifurcation of the spinal cord to which the septum was very closely adherent. Seven years later she has a normally valgoid foot without spasticity and her left plantar response is still extensor.

Case 62, aged 17 months at time of operation, had spasticity of both lower limbs. Seven years later his spasticity is much reduced and he has good voluntary control of his hips. There is no sensory loss and he has normal bladder and bowel control. At laminectomy he was found to have an enlarged terminal spinal cord which has been classified as myelodysplasia. It is possible that the decompression resulting from the operation may account for his improvement but there was no extrinsic abnormality which could be dealt with surgically.

Case 95, aged 44 years at the time of operation, was incontinent and had had two unsuccessful bladder operations in the hope of improving this. She also had increasing weakness of the whole left lower limb which necessitated her wearing an iron. Two years post-operatively she has much better leg function and no longer wears irons. There has been no change in her bladder control and because of ascending urinary infection she has had to have a ureteric diversion performed. Follow-up is short because she has emigrated. At laminectomy she was found to have an intramedullary dermoid in the conus medullaris and among the cauda equina. It was possible to remove the cyst completely.

IMPROVED (34 CASES)

Cases regarded as improved are grouped according to their pre-operative main symptoms: incontinence, unilateral sensory changes, unilateral pes cavovarus, monoplegia and paraplegia.

Incontinence (7 cases)

The cases in this group were all totally incontinent by the definition given in Chapter 16.

Three cases, including 1 adult, recovered normal urinary control, but the adult's advantage was short-term because she had chronic urinary infection and later hydronephrosis necessitating ureteric diversion and cystectomy. This patient had a lumbosacral lipoma continuous with the filum terminale. Of the 2 children, 1 aged 10 years had a meningocele manqué with recurrent nerve roots and adhesions of the right cauda equina, the other aged $9\frac{1}{2}$ years had diastematomyelia with a septum and adherent nerves recurrent from the spinal cord (3–5 years follow-up).

The other 4 cases all improved in some respect. Cases 25 (adult) and 76 (boy aged 5 years) both lack complete urinary control but have recovered sensation so that they are aware that the bladder is full and can act accordingly; they no longer suffer continual wetting. The adult had a lumbosacral lipoma continuous with the filum terminale, and the boy had a meningocele manqué. Case 83, a girl aged 9 years, now has a normal bladder but continues to have neurogenic equinovarus with sensory loss and trophic ulceration. She had diastematomyelia without septum, with multiple adhesions and aberrant nerve roots (4–7 years follow-up).

The final case (23) was aged 3 years at the time of operation and during the next 7 years has recovered from continual urinary leakage to good control except occasionally at night. This improvement might be ascribed to her growing older but her anal reflex is present on the right side and absent on the left with corresponding perianal sensory loss; her knee and ankle jerks continue to be absent and her plantar responses are flexor. At operation she was found to have intrathecal bands and light adhesions which we considered at the time as being of no significance but they were removed from the terminal spinal cord; microscopy showed them to be only very small blood vessels.

Unilateral sensory changes (8 cases)

Of 6 cases with trophic ulceration, all but 1 have required subsequent local surgery, principally because of residual infection but also because of foot deformity causing undue pressure when wearing

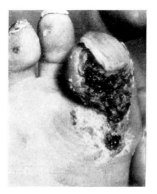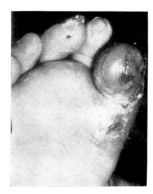

Figure 19.1: Case 26. Trophic lesion of great toe immediately before (left) *and 6 weeks after operation* (right)

shoes. In most of them the area of sensory loss has been slightly reduced but in only 1 of them, Case 21, has there been complete recovery of skin sensation; this is the one who has had no further trophic manifestation, she had diastematomyelia without a septum but with traction bands. Three cases had diastematomyelia with a septum, in 2 of them the septum was causing pressure, very slightly in Case 6 but severely in Case 14; in the third there were traction bands (Case 30). In Cases 26 and 100 there were traction abnormalities; in the former (*Figures 19.1, 19.2*) from a subcutaneous lipoma attaching directly to neural tissue and in the latter, multiple bands of meningocele manqué type.

Cases 7 and 32 have both recovered vibration sense and reflexes. In both cases there was diastematomyelia without a septum but with traction bands.

Case 100 has been followed for $2\frac{1}{2}$ years and the rest have all been followed for between 7 and 13 years.

Unilateral pes cavovarus (7 cases)

As already mentioned, foot deformity once established in the child is likely to get worse and 2 of these cases have required subsequent orthopaedic treatment.

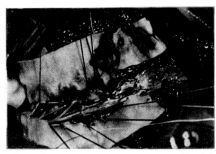

Cranial   Caudal

(a) *Dura mater opened. Subcutaneous tissue and its fibrous continuation to the dura being retracted; extradural continuation of the band passes behind the two central stay sutures. Retracted dura mater reflects the light strongly and appears convex, although it is actually concave. Band is seen again to the left of the retracted dura fanning out intrathecally to be attached to the conus medullaris (Sv1). The filum terminale is running in the midline in the centre of the field but passes towards the right in the right part of the field*

(b) *At end of operation. Fibrous band has been divided at its points of attachment which are seen projecting from the spinal cord just to the left of centre of the field. To right of centre, cut end of filum terminale and the gap produced by its retraction are clearly shown. Original point of attachment is the blackened area seen at the caudal end of the dural opening*

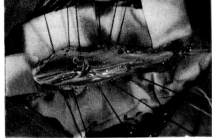

Cranial   Caudal

Figure 19.2: Case 26

Case 73 had a lateral popliteal palsy which partially recovered, leaving some muscular incoordination which required tendon transplants 2 years after laminectomy, and there has been no change in the following 5 years. Case 54 continued to have a tendency to get sores because of persistent valgus of his toes and they have all been amputated; in the 3 years following laminectomy he recovered control of his bladder and continues to have control a further 4 years later. Each case had a tight filum terminale associated with adhesions of the cauda equina.

In the other 5 cases foot deformity ceased, no further surgery has been required and areas of sensory loss or reflexes have improved.

Four had diastematomyelia; in Case 9 a septum was causing lateral pressure and in Cases 12, 24 and 44 there were traction bands but no septum. Case 10 had a band (a nerve) passing from a neural arch through the dura mater to attach to the spinal cord on which it was clearly dragging. Follow-up was from 5 to 10 years.

Monoplegia (7 cases)

All the cases of monoplegia had unilateral foot abnormalities but associated with either paralysis or spasticity. In every case there was improvement either in the spasticity or of power. All but 1 have recovered good foot action but 2 of them required orthopaedic operations; Case 8 had an elongation of the heel cord and Case 69 correction of hallux valgus. The single exception, Case 13, required stabilization of his foot owing to deformity; in his case the filum terminale was found to be adherent laterally and although the adhesions were freed, it was so tight that it needed to be divided. Case 8 had a traction and pressure lesion from a transverse band in the dura, adherent and pressing on the terminal spinal cord as well as having additional bands. The remainder all had traction lesions from bands and adhesions, in Case 61 associated with a lumbosacral lipoma. Follow-up was from 5 to 10 years.

Paraplegia (5 cases)

In every case of paraplegia the element of spasticity has disappeared.

Case 2, aged $14\frac{1}{2}$ years, was almost flail at the time of laminectomy but has recovered good voluntary muscle function proximally in the lower limbs but he wears a caliper on one leg; he has bladder sensation but little control. He very much enjoys playing football in leisure time but has sustained two fractures as the result of continuing sensory loss. He had a transverse pressure band in his dura mater at Lv1 level which was severely constricting the spinal cord. The conus medullaris was over the body of Lv3. Follow-up was for 13 years.

Case 31, aged 8 years, has recovered good voluntary control of both lower limbs but has required transplantation of the hamstring muscles from the tibia to the back of the femur on each side and no longer uses calipers. His bladder control is very much improved. He had a large dermoid cyst with considerable adhesions to the cauda equina on both sides. The cyst was emptied; it was not possible to remove it. Follow-up was for 8 years.

Case 70, aged 2 years, has had progressive improvement in control and strength in the lower limbs without foot deformity. Her bladder control is normal but she is still liable to recurrent cystitis. She had a dermoid cyst in the spinal cord which was emptied by aspiration. Follow-up was for 6 years.

Case 75, aged 19 years, presented with bilateral popliteal palsy and incontinence. All his foot muscles have recovered and he walks normally. Before laminectomy he had recurrent septic lesions on his left foot and the fourth toe had been amputated. There has been a little improvement in his bladder control. He had diastematomyelia without a septum but with arachnoiditis and adhesions of the spinal cord dorsally in the region of the diastematomyelia. It was possible to free the spinal cord at laminectomy. Follow-up was for 5 years.

Case 91, aged 18 months, presented with generalized weakness of the trunk and lower limbs and a left foot-drop. At laminectomy from Cv6 to Tv6, in which region there were laminal defects, extensive hydromyelia was found. The cyst was very thin walled and it was opened. In the 4 years following operation he has developed normal musculature although he still has a high dorsal kyphos. There is slight cavovarus deformity in the left foot but this is well used. He was totally incontinent before operation but now has good control. It is in the nature of this condition that this good progress may not last.

Subject Index

Index of Case Histories

Numbers in italics denote pages with illustrations.

INDEX OF CASE HISTORIES